Food for Fitness After Fifty:

*A Menu for Good Health
in the Later Years*

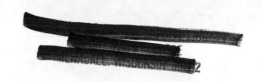

FOOD
for
FITNESS
After
FIFTY:

*A Menu
for Good Health
in the Later Years*

Fredrick J. Stare, MD

Virginia Aronson, RD, MS
Department of Nutrition
Harvard University

George F. Stickley Company
210 West Washington Square
Philadelphia, PA 19106

Introduction

Dr. Daniel Ruge
Physician to the President

When Ronald Reagan made his second Presidential victory speech on election night in November of 1984, he explained with a chuckle, "Good habits are hard to break." Politics aside, this motto can certainly serve us all as a key to healthful living. Fortunately, it is never too late to adopt sensible health habits.

Good food and good health go hand in hand—from life's first beginnings to the ripest years of the longest life span. Unfortunately, the real health concerns of the long-lived population have often been ignored in favor of required medical treatment for age-related ills and the ever-popular but highly questionable "cure-alls." Preventive health care should be an essential component of the older person's lifestyle, so that the tendency to seek outside therapy (i.e., over-the-counter drugs, supplements and "miracle" products) can be reduced. And the attainment and maintenance of optimal fitness can help enormously in the prevention or delay of age-related diseases, thereby minimizing the need for therapeutic intervention.

Despite the abundance of "health" claims which bombard us daily from newsstands, magazine covers, billboards, radio and television, and the marketplace in general, it is not possible for Americans to purchase fitness in the same way they are able to buy nearly everything else. Yet, stocking up on nutrition knowledge and fitness facts *can* assist health-conscious consumers in adopting a healthful lifestyle. All that is required is a general understanding of nutrition basics, the motivation to make the lifestyle changes that promote physical fitness, and the willingness to spend the time and energy required to live a long and healthy life. When one examines the alternatives, the decision to live well is an easy one!

The foundation of a long life is partly structured from years of sound dietary habits and regular physical activity. As a physician, I have received no formal training in nutrition and exercise physiology, but have long advocated the importance of sensible eating habits and physical activity—*at all ages.* This book can serve as an excellent resource for those individuals over age fifty who plan to enjoy a long, healthy life. The nutritionists/authors provide readers with easy-to-read guidelines to balancing the diet, controlling body weight, starting an exercise program, dealing with some of the common ills of aging, and enjoying a healthful diet. After all, Dr. Stare (at age 74) is a living example of the success of good health habits, and his young coauthor plans to follow suit!

In an era fraught with fitness fads and diet gimmicks, it is encouraging to discover common sense, factual advice on nutrition for older Americans. And for those of us who are over the age of fifty, it is especially encouraging to be able to turn to a trustworthy source of self-health information. Although we may not be world leaders or even youthful aspirers, it is not too late for *any* of us to become active members of the movement to optimal health.

Contents

Ronald Reagan: A Healthy Appetite for Politics—and Life!

President Ronald Reagan is quite a bit over the age of fifty, but his youthful level of fitness certainly does not reflect this: a combination of sensible diet, regular exercise, and stimulating environments serves to keep Reagan fit 'n firm. With the stress which accompanies one of the most demanding jobs in today's world, Reagan is one senior citizen who cannot let poor health jeopardize his—and our—future.

According to Dr. Daniel Ruge, Mr. Reagan's former physician, "The President has always been a very moderate and healthy man with a love for the outdoors. His breakfasts consist of cereal, with an egg on alternate days, fruit in some form, toast or muffin and decaffeinated coffee. Lunches are made up of a large variety of soups, there are also frequent salads and ice cream occasionally. He likes macaroni and cheese, hamburgers, and lasagna; below are some of his dinner menus selected at random:

October 5—Boiled beef, horseradish sauce, selection of garden vegetables, Hominy Royale, Boston lettuce and alfalfa sprout salad, warm apple tart.

October 8—Turkey breast scaloppini with nutty herb filling, green noodles, sautéed yellow squash, Romaine lettuce, blue cheese dressing, lemon sorbet.

September 27—Boneless chicken roulade, lemon/caper sauce, crispy broccoli sesame, matchstick potatoes with leeks, Bibb lettuce with chives, radish dressing, pears gratinées, Chablis wine sauce.

"I have had nothing to do with the President's exercise program, and have had very little to do with his diet. In fact, I try to take tips from him!"

According to Reagan's own report:

"Exercise comes pretty naturally to me, since I've done it my entire life. When I was younger, I was a lifeguard during the summers, and I played football in high school and college. And for all of my adult life, I have enjoyed horseback riding and working outdoors.

Over the years, I have learned that one key to exercise is to find something you enjoy. The other key is to keep the exercise varied.

In my view, every exercise program should have an outdoor element to it—whether jogging, bicycling, skiing, hiking or walking. I prefer horseback riding and, whenever possible, hard manual labor.

The other component of my exercise program is geared toward the indoors. There is not a lot of wood to chop or trails to clear on the White House lawn, so I have set up a gym on the second floor. My calisthenic and gym routine actually started as therapy after the shooting, but the doctors say I am now in better shape than when I came to the White House.

My program, which was designed by a professional, consists of 10 minutes of warm-up calisthenics, aimed at limbering up specific muscles, followed by about 15 minutes of workout on the machines. I have two different sets of exercises I do on alternate days. Each exercise is for specific muscles.

Most people have a problem sticking to their exercise routine because they get bored. The beauty of the routine I follow is (1) the alternate sets of exercises, which give some variety, and (2) the brevity of the routines, which gets me out of there in half an hour. And I have come up with a few tricks of my own. I have a TV in front of the treadmill so that when I'm walking, I can also watch the news. Of course, because of the responsibility of this job, work and travel break up the routine enough that I can exercise regularly, yet without it becoming monotonous." (PARADE Magazine, Dec. 4, 1983)

At 6'1", President Reagan is a trim 190 pounds. His sensible lifestyle patterns exclude cigarette smoking and immoderate alcohol consumption, while encouraging adequate rest and relaxation. Finding time for "R & R" was illustrated by a newspaper reporter in the sports pages during the President's first term:

"He came into the press box in the second inning, carrying two Cokes and two bags of peanuts. There was a thin layer of sweat on the brow of Ronald Reagan, President of the United States.

'You won't believe the traffic out there,' he said last night at the first game of the World Series. 'That stuff is backed up all the way to the Beltway.'" (Leigh Montville, *Boston Globe*, Oct. 12, 1983)

From the White House to Camp David to the ballpark, President Reagan sets a healthy example for people of all ages: Eat moderately, exercise regularly, and enjoy life. No doubt he will be around to enjoy many more years of good health and political activity!

Part I

Appetizers: Basic Nutrition Concepts

APPETIZERS: BASIC NUTRITION CONCEPTS

Does the following menu look familiar to you?

Breakfast: Toast with jelly, coffee or tea
Lunch: Soup and crackers
Teatime: Tea and cookies
Supper: Tuna or chicken salad sandwich
Bedtime: Cocoa and cookies

If variations on this menu constitute your current diet, don't think you're alone. Too many older adults follow a bland, repetitious, and not very nutritious dietary pattern similar to that given above. Reasons vary, but most elderly individuals blame their poor diets on poor income, health status, social situation, and mental attitude. It is the last drawback which can so easily be altered to result in a healthful diet, a healthy lifestyle, and a long and happy lifetime.

Your later years can be thought of simply as the extension of your earlier years, but with the emergence of different physical and emotional features. The degree to which the process of aging will influence your overall health status depends on individual nutrition throughout the life span. But even when adulthood is in full swing and the last revolutions of the life cycle are underway, what you eat still affects how you feel.

By the time you reach your "golden years," individual lifestyle patterns will have been established, and certain habits may have become ingrained. Diet can prove to be difficult to alter at this late date, especially if poor health and/or social isolation are allowed to detract from the overall quality of life. However, it is important for you to attempt to meet the nutritional needs of your aging body in order to maximize your individual potential for health and longevity.

Even though the expected life spans for men and women have not increased significantly during this century, the doors are now open to live your life to its fullest for a myriad of years. In order to enjoy a lifetime which is of suitable quality, however, you need to remain healthy. Proper nutrition and a well-balanced diet play integral roles in the achievement and maintenance of a favorable health status and an optimal level of well-being . . . at any age.

If your diet is not well-balanced early in life, you may experience the undesirable after-effects later on, during your adult years and into your senior citizen days—if you live long enough, that is. Since adulthood should be a time for substantial goal achievement— marriage, child-bearing, parenting, career advancement, property ownership, financial investment, retirement—interference due to physical and mental impairment needs to be minimized. If you are well-

3

nourished during infancy, childhood, adolescence and early adulthood, your dietary intake should continue to be supportive of favorable health. But even if you enter your "golden years" with a history of improper nutrition, it is not too late to develop the healthy eating habits which can enhance vitality and promote longevity.

So why not develop a healthy mental attitude, right NOW? Contrary to popular belief, you *can* teach an old dog new tricks! With your diet, the trick is simply to apply some basic nutrition concepts.

THE BASIC NUTRIENTS

What is "nutrition"?

Nutrition is the science of food and its relation to physical and psychological health. Nutrition deals with how the body uses the food we eat to produce energy to keep warm and move about, to build tissues and maintain smooth function. Nutrition provides us with eating satisfaction as well, because food is certainly one of life's pleasures.

Nutrition is to the body what auto service is to a car: if you provide your car with regular refueling, see that it gets regular check-ups and repairs, it will run smoothly and take you where you want to go. This is also true for your body: if you fuel yourself with the proper diet of the basic nutrients, you can have the energy and good health to go wherever you want to go. Supported by regular medical check-ups and maintenance as needed, your body will last you a lifetime—a long and healthy one at that, and far longer than that of your car.

Obviously, nutrition plays an essential role in overall health care, from the day you are conceived into your later years. Although major dietary changes are probably not required (unless prescribed by your physician), by improving the general nature of your diet, you may be able to enhance the quality of your life. Eat OK—Feel OK! Eat better, Feel better!

What is a nutrient?

A nutrient is a specific substance, a chemical, that is required by living organisms—plants or animals—for growth and maintenance of life. There are some 50 known nutrients which fit into six major categories: carbohydrate, protein, fat, vitamins, minerals and water.

All of these nutrients are chemicals and all are found in the foods we eat. Yet, no one food, not even human milk, contains all of the essential nutrients in adequate amounts. Hence, to obtain all of these nutrients—and no doubt others yet unknown—eating a wide variety of different foods is essential.

Carbohydrates

How do you define "carbohydrate"?

A carbohydrate is a chemical compound composed only of carbon, oxygen and hydrogen. The carbohydrates that are nutrients include a variety of sugars and starches. The "simple sugars" include sucrose or "table sugar," generally obtained from sugar cane or beets, fructose, the common sugar of honey and some fruits, and lactose, the sugar naturally present in milk. Maltose is a less common sugar which is found in malt products.

Edible starches occur mainly in cereals and in tubers such as potatoes, and they differ structurally from sugars in that they are more "complex," but are also composed only of carbon, oxygen and hydrogen.

Sugars and starches are the main source of calories in our diets, providing approximately half of our total calories. When digested, all sugars and starches are broken down into a simpler sugar called glucose which is the type of sugar that occurs in the blood—blood sugar—and which nourishes all body cells.

Fiber is also a carbohydrate, but is poorly digested by the human digestive system, so it provides few calories. Fiber is not a nutrient itself, but is essential in the diet mainly because it provides bulk in the lower intestine to help in elimination and in preventing constipation.

Good food sources of carbohydrates include fruits, vegetables, whole grain and enriched breads and cereals, milk and milk products. Although sweets high in sugar such as ice cream, cookies, or pie may not be the lowest calorie sources of carbohydrates, such foods can provide carbohydrate and other nutrients along with eating enjoyment.

Are carbohydrates as fattening as they say?

Carbohydrates are less fattening than "they" say, the "they" being people not very well informed about nutrition. To become overweight, fat, or even obese, one must—over a period of time that can be many weeks, months, or years—consume more calories than are needed to maintain a reasonable body weight.

All foods provide calories as well as nutrients. Carbohydrates and proteins each provide the same number of calories per unit of weight— 4 calories per gram (about 115 per ounce). Fat provides a little more than twice that amount, 9 calories per gram (about 260 per ounce). Alcohol, although generally not considered a food, provides about 7 calories per gram; since alcoholic beverages are consumed with growing frequency, alcohol must be considered in the total caloric intake of many people.

Thus, fats and alcohol are actually more fattening than carbohydrates when considered in equal amounts. Since we generally put butter or margarine on our bread and potatoes, and frequently sour cream on the latter, we may find that the bread and potatoes, which are full of carbohydrates, are only "fattening" because we consume them with generous quantities of fat. So, don't blame the carbohydrates for being "fattening"! Blame yourself for adding on all those fat-calories. Diets *high* in carbohydrates but *low* in fats are generally less conducive to poor health—including overweight.

Protein

Where do we get protein?

The main protein foods for most of us are meat, fish, and poultry, but we also obtain protein from legumes (peas and beans), nuts, eggs, milk and milk products and cereals. In fact, in the quantities that cereals are consumed, particularly in the rest of the world, more people get more protein from cereals than from any other source.

Protein is composed of amino acids, about 22 of them. Somewhat less than half of the amino acids are called "essential" amino acids, that is, they must be obtained from the foods we eat because they cannot be made in our body tissues. The remaining 10 or 12 amino acids are called "nonessential" because if we do not get them in sufficient quantities in the food we eat, we can make them in our body tissues, particularly in the liver.

All animal proteins (except collagen) contain all of the essential amino acids. All other sources of protein—nuts, legumes, and cereals for example—are lacking or low in one or more essential amino acids, but are generous sources of the nonessential ones. Thus, most meals are better from a nutritional viewpoint if they contain at least a small amount of animal protein—meat, fish, poultry, milk, yogurt, cheese, or egg—to supply all of the essential amino acids.

Americans tend to consume too much animal protein, however, usually taking in at least twice the amount of protein needed daily by the body. Therefore, since it is so easy to obtain an adequate amount of this nutrient, you need not fear protein malnutrition if you fail to consume 10 ounces of steak for dinner! Your body is most likely getting an adequate, if not too generous, amount of dietary protein.

Can a vegetarian still obtain adequate protein?

Yes, with proper planning and special attention to menu design, vegetarians can balance their diets to include the protein they require. Strict vegetarians ("vegans") do not eat any animal products, so their diets exclude milk, cheese, yogurt, and eggs as well as meat, poultry, and fish, which can cause a protein deficiency. For those who do include some animal foods, this undesirable imbalance can be easily avoided.

Foods of animal origin contain high-quality protein because adequate amounts of all of the essential amino acids are present. Plant products, however, are low or deficient in one or more of the essential amino acids. Therefore, the protein is incomplete and not of high nutritional quality.

In order to compensate for this inadequacy, small amounts of animal protein should be eaten along with plant foods: Have a glass of milk with your peanut butter sandwich, melt some cheese on your steamed broccoli spears, and mix some chopped egg into your vegetable-rice casserole.

Plant foods can also be eaten in specific combinations so that their specific amino acid inadequacies are compensated for. For example, wheat bread is low in the amino acid lysine, but peanuts are not; hence, a peanut butter sandwich contains protein of improved nutritional quality. These are called "complementary" protein foods. Use the chart below to assist in keeping your protein intake complementary.

Complementary Foods—Easy Reference Chart

Plant Foods ←—————————→ Animal Foods
(meat, poultry, fish,
eggs, cheese, milk,
yogurt)

Legumes ←—————————→ Grains
(dried beans and peas)
(barley, buckwheat,
corn, oats, millet, rice,
rye, wheat)

Legumes ←—————————→ Nuts
Legumes ←—————————→ Seeds

Note: Strict vegetarian diets—that is, without any animal protein—can also be inadequate in nutrients other than essential amino acids, including iron, calcium, riboflavin, and vitamin B_{12}. It is best to obtain individualized diet counseling from a registered dietitian or other nutrition professional if you adhere to such a restrictive regime.

Fat

Do we need to eat fat at all?

Yes, we need to eat some fat in order to obtain adequate amounts of the essential fatty acid known as linoleic acid. Fats are classified chemically as *saturated* and *unsaturated*, and the latter into mono- and polyunsaturated. Fats, as they occur in foods, are mixtures of saturated and unsaturated fatty acids in varying proportions. For example, most animal fats have generous amounts of saturated and monounsaturated fats and small amounts of polyunsaturated fats; common vegetable oils such as soy, corn, safflower, and sunflower oils have generous amounts of polyunsaturated fatty acids, moderate amounts of monounsaturated, and small amounts of saturated fats. However, there are two vegetable oils—coconut and palm—which are rich in saturated fats.

Foods high in fat may be easily identified, (such as butter, lard, margarine, marbled meats, cream, and fried foods), or these items can be "sneaky" sources of "hidden" fat. Some common sources of invisible fat include nuts, whole milk and whole milk cheeses, high fat meats (like bacon, sausage, luncheon meats, duck and goose), salad dressings, sour cream, cream cheese, olives, and prepared foods which are high in fat content.

In addition to providing the essential fatty acid—linoleic—fats also improve the taste of a meal, and provide "satiety" value since they take longer to digest. Thus, we do need some fat in the diet, enough to provide 30% of total calories, which is at least 5 to 10% less than most of us usually consume.

How fattening IS fat? Does food fat automatically turn into body fat?

How much fat is fattening depends on how much fat—and other sources of calories—are consumed, and on how many calories are expended in the activities of physical work and exercise. All foods, if consumed in excess of the body's needs, can become bodily fat—which is simply the body's method for storing excess calories.

Ordinarily, we consume about 300-400 grams of carbohydrate per day, 130–150 of fat, and 100–120 of protein—for a total of 2500–3000 calories. If we increase the fat by 50% and at the same time decrease our intake of carbohydrate and protein by about the same number of calories, the extra fat is not fattening. But if the extra fat is in addition to our usual intake of carbohydrate, protein, and alcohol, then the extra fat *is* fattening. This, of course, assumes that our energy expenditure (physical activity) remains the same.

Since fat is such a concentrated source of calories, and because it can be hidden in many foodstuffs, an intake of too many fat-calories can occur all too easily. Because a diet lower in fat is generally better for one's health—as well as figure—those foods high in fat may be best kept to a minimum.

Are some kinds of fat preferable to others?

In general, overall reduction in fat intake is a wise idea for most Americans. We tend to eat just too much of it—and it shows, on our bulging waistlines and in our fat-clogged arteries. However, in the latter regard, certain types of fat are less desirable than others.

Saturated fat tends to elevate blood cholesterol levels, whereas the unsaturated fats do not. Therefore, nutritionists advise consumers to emphasize the less saturated forms of fat when choosing to include fat in their diets: this means margarine instead of butter; vegetable oils like soy, corn, sunflower and safflower instead of animal fats, shortening, lard, or the more saturated coconut and palm oils; and fish, lean poultry, and non-animal proteins in place of meats.

Thus, if your diet is relatively high in fat, that is, fat makes up over 35% of your total caloric intake, it is best to reduce your overall fat intake. Those fats you do include should be those high in the polyunsaturated fats, notably the above-mentioned vegetable oils, with less of the fats rich in monosaturated (such as olive oil, peanut oil, nuts) and even less of the highly saturated animal fats, coconut oil, and palm oil. And since fats are often "hidden" in processed foods, especially the highly stable coconut/palm oils, you can start fat-watching by reading the nutrient information and ingredient lists on the labels of the foods you buy.

Is cholesterol another kind of fat?

Cholesterol is not "another kind of fat." Chemically, it is a "higher alcohol." Not that you will get "high" on it, but it is a little more complicated (or higher) in its chemical structure than ethanol, which is the alcohol in alcoholic beverages (too much of which will make one "high").

However, cholesterol is found only in animal tissue and always in association with fat. Thus, there is no cholesterol in olive, corn or soybean oils because these are oils of vegetable origin. Yet there is cholesterol in egg yolk, meat fat, butter, and whole milk and cheeses made from it because these are of animal origin.

However, we also make cholesterol in several body tissues, particularly in the liver. Cholesterol is an essential body substance (not a nutrient) and is needed to make vitamin D and several of the sex hormones. When we consume less cholesterol, our body tissue makes a little more—but usually not enough more to make up for what we have eliminated via dietary changes.

Egg yolk (not the white) is by far the single most important source of food cholesterol in the American diet. Liver and other organ meats are also rich sources of cholesterol, but they are not consumed as frequently by most of us as are eggs. Certain shellfish such as shrimp also contribute cholesterol, but not too many of us can say that we overindulge on seafood with any regularity.

Should I eliminate eggs and liver, just to be extra careful?

No! You need not eliminate eggs or liver to be "extra careful." However, if your physician thinks your blood cholesterol is a little higher than he would like it to be, *and* you have some of the other "risk factors" of heart disease such as a history in your family of early death (before age 65) from heart disease, a blood pressure that is moderately elevated, if you are a cigarette smoker, overweight, have diabetes, and are not very active physically—you might well try to lower your cholesterol. The best way to try to do this is by taking off any extra pounds and reducing intake of saturated fat and egg yolks to 2–3 a week. If you consume liver or other organ meats often, it would be best to limit this to once a week or less.

Vitamins

How many vitamins do I need?

Altogether, there are 13 vitamins known to be essential to human growth and health. Nutritionists separate these "essential" vitamins into two categories: those soluble in water and those which are soluble in fat. Because of their specific chemical properties, these two categories function differently in the body. Also, the water-soluble vitamins in general are not stored appreciably, while the fat-soluble vitamins can be stored in body fat depots.

The water-soluble vitamins include the 8 B-vitamins (also called the B-complex) and vitamin C or ascorbic acid. The four fat-soluble vitamins are A, D, E, and K. All of these vitamins are available in our food supply, but we tend to get much of our D from the action of sunlight on the skin. The chart below provides a list of the essential vitamins, bodily functions, and best food sources, as well as potential dangers associated with taking in excessive amounts of these important but certainly not harmless nutrients.

There are so many different vitamins to keep track of, why not make it easier by taking a daily vitamin supplement?

True, there are many vitamins, but vitamin supplements seldom contain all of them in the quantities thought to be necessary. Thus, a daily vitamin replacement is not likely to provide all of the vitamins you need in the desirable amounts. It is wiser to obtain the vitamins—and

Major Function In:

Vitamin	Energy	Body Cells	Body Processes	Symptoms of Overdose
A		Increases resistance to infection	Maintains normal skin; promotes healthy eyes and eye adaptation in dim light; aids growth	Yellow deposits on hands and feet, retarded growth, dry skin, headaches, bone pain, lack of appetite, hair loss, liver damage, death
B_1 (Thiamin), B_2 (Riboflavin) & Niacin	Aids in energy use		Promote healthy skin, eyes, nerves, appetite and digestion	Flushing and itching skin, skin disorders, liver damage, peptic ulcer, high blood sugar levels, gout
C		Strengthens blood vessels; speeds wound healing; increases resistance to infection	Aids in iron use	Gastrointestinal disturbances, kidney disorders, damage to growing bones, rebound scurvy (swollen gums, loose teeth), muscle pain
D			Promotes bone development	Retarded physical and mental development, nausea, weakness, weight loss, kidney stones, kidney failure, high blood pressure, calcium deposits in tissue, death
E		Antioxidant: protects cell structure in body (also retards food spoilage)		Headaches, nausea, fatigue, blurred vision, inflammation of mouth, intestinal disturbances, muscle weakness, low blood sugar levels, interference with absorption of vitamin K
K			Promotes proper blood clotting	Increased clotting (especially dangerous with certain antidote medications)
B_6 (Pyridoxine)		Involved in protein synthesis		Interferes with certain medications; nerve damage with prolonged use
Folic Acid		Forms red blood cells	Prevents anemia	Masks certain anemias; kidney damage.
B_{12}		Involved in blood formation	Promotes growth, health of nervous system	Liver damage

the many other nutrients you need—from food. And how much more pleasant and tasty a way to obtain them!

It is important to be aware of the clever marketing strategies used to promote the many brands of vitamin supplements available in "health food" stores, pharmacies, even department stores in your area. Door-to-door vitamin sales personnel, in fact, will promote the need for "vitamin insurance" to prevent against or overcome marginal vitamin deficiencies due to modern day living.

Other vitamin sales hype includes claims of curative properties for every ailment from baldness and impotence to senility and irritability, or even cancer, arthritis, and heart disease. By realizing that such claims are merely sales pitches to obtain your money under false pretenses, you can avoid wasting your finances on unnecessary vitamin supplements. And since certain vitamins taken in large doses can prove harmful, alert consumers can protect their health as well as their finances.

Are "natural" vitamins preferable to the synthetic brands?

Absolutely not. Vitamins are specific chemical compounds and are identical in chemical structure and physiological action, whether they are made by nature or by a chemist and produced in huge amounts in a chemical factory. The so-called synthetic preparations are much less expensive, yet the "natural" brands often contain synthetic ingredients as binders and filler, and some actually contain synthetic vitamins to achieve the potency on the label.

Most elderly people short-change themselves of which vitamins?

Many consume diets with less than adequate amounts of vitamins D, A, C, and sometimes thiamin. If the typical older adult continues to eat a varied diet and includes one or two glasses of milk with added vitamin D (skimmed or low-fat milk, fortified with both vitamins A and D), a regular intake of foods high in vitamin A (such as bright yellow and leafy green vegetables), a good source of vitamin C (like a daily orange or glass of orange or other citrus juice, some tomatoes or tomato juice) and whole grain or enriched breads and cereals, vitamin short-changing can be avoided.

Should elderly people take in more vitamins as they get older? And do we need even more under stress?

Aging itself does not increase one's need for vitamins and neither does stress, but both aging and stress have become gimmicks used to sell extra amounts of vitamins to those getting along in years and to those under stress—which includes just about everybody!

Minerals

How many minerals do I need?

You need all of the 21 or so minerals known to be necessary for good nutrition. These include the macrominerals, those present in the body in amounts exceeding 5 grams—still a very small quantity—and the microminerals, available in even lesser quantities. The major or macrominerals include calcium, phosphorus, chloride, potassium, sulphur, sodium, and magnesium, while the trace elements or microminerals now known are iron, manganese, copper, iodine, zinc, cobalt, chromium, fluoride, selenium, and molybdenum, plus nickel, silicon, tin and vanadium. Fortunately, you need not swallow handfuls of mineral pills, but you can get these and the many other nutrients in adequate amounts by eating a varied diet. NOTE: Minerals that may be on the low side, or even deficient, in those adults getting along in years, include calcium (usually because of not consuming enough milk), iron (from meat intakes that are too skimpy and avoidance of leafy greens), and fluoride for those living in a community where the water supply has not been adjusted in the mineral nutrient fluoride to a level of one part per million, a process called fluoridation.

We usually think of fluoride only in connection with lessening tooth decay in children, and in this connection it is most important. A child who has access to fluoridated water from birth to adulthood will have about 70% less tooth decay. But fluoride may also be important at the other end of the spectrum, in slowing down or even preventing the development of osteoporosis, a bone-thinning disease all too common in older Americans. There are few good food sources of fluoride, and in much of our country, small amounts of fluoride have to be added to the water supplies to provide amounts adequate for good health.

If sodium is an essential mineral, why has it received such bad press lately?

Sodium is an essential and a most important mineral. Our principal source of sodium is salt added to foods and used in preparing them, but most foods naturally contain a certain amount of sodium as well. Most people like the taste of salt, which is an acquired taste—and many are consuming far more than the body requires. For most people, an intake of extra sodium is not harmful, so long as the kidneys are functioning well and blood pressure is normal.

The "bad press" sodium has received in recent years is largely due to the fact that about 20% of the American population is prone to high blood pressure (hypertension), and of that 20%, about one-third may help to lower their blood pressure with a reduction in sodium intake. However, this reduction must be quite severe: by as much as 80 to 90%!

With such a reduction, few people find meals tasty, and still fewer can adhere to such a diet plan for very long. Most can do so only under close medical supervision, usually as hospital in-patients.

A recent Commissioner of the FDA fostered considerable bad publicity about salt as a "killer," urging the food industry into developing a number of new low-sodium foods. Such foods are perfectly acceptable as another line of foods to market, and can help to reduce sodium intake as part of a general moderation in salt consumption. However, advertising implications that these products actually serve to lower blood pressure and/or prevent the development of hypertension are quite misleading. Take all such promises with a grain of salt!

So how much sodium do we need?

Most adults consume 5 to 6 grams of sodium (equivalent to 12–14 grams of salt), and we probably need no more than 0.4 to 0.5 grams (1 to 1-1/2 grams of salt). In round numbers, about one third of our usual sodium intake is naturally present in a varied diet, another third is added to our foods in processing, and the final third comes from what we add ourselves in cooking and at the table. If you wish to be prudent about sodium intake, give away your salt shakers and go easy on the salt you use in cooking. Try the many herbs and spices available—make cooking a salt-free taste adventure!

Which foods are especially high in sodium?

Many grain foods are quite high in sodium, and this food group provides us with much of our total sodium intake: breads, cereals (especially quick-cooking brands), biscuits and baked goods all contain leavening agents high in sodium. Milk and processed cheeses contain significant amounts of sodium, as do canned vegetables, certain frozen vegetables, even some fresh vegetables (such as celery, beets, tomatoes) and vegetable juices. Even meat has some sodium—quite a lot, in fact, when smoked, dried, or cured as with bacon, corned beef, hot dogs and luncheon meats, sausages, and ham. Other foods requiring salt in preparation are high in sodium, notably higher than those with significant "natural" sodium contents: olives, soups, bouillon, condiments, pickles and other brined items such as sauerkraut, as well as the items obviously salted to meet our snack cravings such as crackers, pretzels, nuts and chips—for which unsalted varieties are now readily available. Read labels carefully to determine whether specially marked products are indeed low in sodium content and are worth the increased costs.

Why should we emphasize high-potassium foods?

Foods high in potassium such as bananas, oranges, strawberries, dried fruits, potatoes, milk, oatmeal, and many vegetables—especially the dark green leafy choices—should be emphasized in the diets of those who take diuretics, medicines that increase urination to rid the body of excess sodium. Most diuretics also cause loss of potassium which may interfere with the regular rhythm of the heart, and this undesirable side effect can usually be prevented by increasing the intake of foods rich in potassium. If the diet is unable to replace the depleted potassium, a potassium supplement may be prescribed.

Populations which adhere to high-potassium diets are less prone to suffer from hypertension, according to research studies. Although still in the early stages of study, it is believed that a high ratio of potassium to sodium in the diet may exert a protective effect against high blood pressure.

What does calcium intake have to do with dietary sodium/potassium?

Like the possible role of potassium in preventing hypertension, calcium is under research as another mineral nutrient of special benefit in our diets. Since high-calcium foods are also beneficial in prevention against osteoporosis, a diet which emphasizes low-fat milk and milk products may offer you double-barreled protection.

Is it advisable to take mineral supplements, just in case?

Mineral supplements should only be taken on the advice of a physician. Commonly, this might be a calcium supplement if one does not consume much milk, an iron supplement if one has a low blood hemoglobin level and hence, a certain degree of iron deficiency anemia, and possibly a fluoride supplement to help delay or even treat osteoporosis.

All of us need fluoride—infants, children, adults, and their elders—in order to help keep calcium fixed in the hard tissues of the body, primarily the teeth and bones. The result is less tooth decay and stronger bones—and as we grow older, possibly less osteoporosis. For those in their later years, this may mean fewer broken bones from minor falls.

Self-prescribed mineral supplements are a waste of money at best, and can lead to nutrient imbalances and undesirable health effects. Like vitamin supplements, most "just in case" urgings for mineral supplementation emanate from those who will make money from your attempts at nutritional "insurance."

What about supplements aimed at older people for that "rundown" feeling?

Generally, that "rundown" feeling refers to an iron deficiency anemia, and the many tonics available to treat that condition are generally various preparations of iron. Some also have added vitamins, but only the iron is potentially effective. Preparations of "iron salts," such as Ferrous Sulfate are equally effective, and much less expensive. Let your physician decide if you need an iron supplement, and if so, he or she can suggest one which is appropriate for your needs (and affordable!). Lack of adequate rest or sleep, stress, and inadequate exercise are also common causes of that "rundown" feeling. Maybe all you need is a brief nap in the afternoon, an extra hour of sleep at night, and a brisk daily walk to give you that "pep" you seek!

Water

Is water actually considered a nutrient?

Yes, water is a nutrient, and a most important one. In fact, one could say it is the most important nutrient because we could live longer without any of the other nutrients and without food than we could survive without water. Some waters, particularly hard waters, are good sources of some mineral nutrients, such as calcium and magnesium. Some waters are also good natural sources of the mineral nutrient fluoride (and of course, all waters can be good sources of fluoride after they have been fluoridated).

How much water do I need to drink every day?

Medically, an adequate water intake is judged by the output of urine. If you put out 1½ to 2 quarts of urine per 24 hours, you are consuming enough water. Remember, coffee, tea, milk, soft drinks, beer or wine, and the juices of fruits and vegetables are good sources of water. Foods also contain considerable amounts of water. Thus, if you drink 6 to 8 glasses of fluid along with the water naturally present in your foods, you should be obtaining an adequate supply of this important nutrient. In humid weather, in poor health/fever, and with heavy exertion, fluid intake needs to be increased, sometimes markedly.

Thirst is *not* an accurate indicator of fluid needs, and older people especially can become dehydrated quite easily.

Note that a significant fluid intake can help to stimulate a sluggish digestive tract, and thus is a boon to those plagued by constipation woes.

Fiber

What also helps a lazy digestive system?

A lazy digestive system can also be aided by an increased fiber intake. This means some bran such as bran-containing cereals, more whole-grain breads and cereals, plus more fruits and vegetables (particularly those in which you ordinarily eat the skins and seeds, such as plums, prunes, grapes, raisins, cucumber, eggplant, and potato). Lazy digestive systems also may function better if they have access to 5 or 6 small meals a day, rather than our usual 2 or 3.

Exercise is an excellent method to strengthen the digestive tract musculature, thereby increasing the efficiency of digestion. This also can help you to work up a thirst, and thereby increase fluid intakes and enhance digestive speed. Only a lazy individual—diet-wise and exercise-wise—suffers from a lazy digestive tract!

Is there anything wrong with using laxatives to help out?

No. Laxatives can be used occasionally, but it is not a good idea to become dependent on these medicinals, because the digestive tract is then not functioning properly on its own. Also, laxative abuse has certain side effects including loss of essential nutrients; the use of such preparations can be taxing financially; and the alternatives are so much healthier: a good consumption of fluids, plenty of fruits, vegetables, and grain foods, regular exercise, and a relaxed lifestyle are far more appealing than taking medicine. If you find that you need a little "natural" help, prune juice has laxative properties, as does methyl cellulose (fiber) sold under trade names as "natural" laxatives.

FOOD GROUPS—THE BASIC FOUR

How can I be sure that my diet includes all of these nutrients? It seems too confusing!

Your diet will include all of the essential nutrients required for good health if based on a varied selection of foods from what are known as the "Basic Four Food Groups."

As an older person, what are the food Groups from the Basic Four on which I need to base my diet?

Your best bet is to emphasize the food groups which are lowest in fat-calories and highest in fiber. This means more choices from the Fruit and Vegetable Group as well as the Bread and Cereal Group, with portion sizes kept moderate since too much of anything can eventually cause caloric overload. The food groups with more fat-calories should receive less emphasis with choices kept to the leaner, low-fat selections. From the Milk and Cheese Group, moderate portions of the skim and low-fat milk products are advisable; as well as modest servings of: lean meat or poultry, fish or eggs, low-fat cottage cheese, and any dried legumes are the best to include from the Meat and Alternates Group.

Other foods—sweets, fats, and alcoholic beverages—are not the items you want to emphasize in your diet, but you need not eliminate these higher calorie products entirely. A moderate amount on an occasional basis of your favorite dessert, a small glass of wine before dinner, even a dollop of sour cream on a baked potato when dining out can add pleasure to your diet without devastating your health. The key, of course, is *moderation*.

The Basic Four Food Groups are the same whether you are an older person, middle-aged, or young—only the portion size differs.

How much do I need to include from each food group?

As you get over age 50—or older—you need to include the outlined number of servings from each group required by an adult, but keep your portion sizes on the small side. This is because your caloric needs are declining gradually as you age, but your *nutritional* requirements will remain relatively stable. By adjusting your serving *sizes*—rather than reducing the *number* of servings or even *eliminating* food groups—you can avoid overdoing it on calories without skimping on your nutrient intake. Weight control is largely a matter of portion control—plus a hefty serving of exercise. But more on that topic in the next chapter.

What does each food group contribute to nutrient intake?

Although each of the food groups contains a variety of foods which contribute different nutrients, each group is noted as a source of specific nutrients: 1) The Fruit and Vegetable Group provides us with vitamins C and A, plus fiber, as well as other vitamins and minerals; 2) the Bread and Cereal Group gives us carbohydrate, fiber, B-vitamins and iron, plus some other vitamins and minerals as well as protein; 3) the Milk and Cheese Group is our best source of calcium, but also contributes riboflavin, protein, other vitamins and minerals; 4) the Meat and Alternates Group is our popular source of high-quality protein, along with iron, B-vitamins, and other minerals. Both of the last two groups add essential fatty acids to the diet, as do other sources such as vegetable oils, margarine, and salad dressings. Put them all together in the form of delicious meals and snacks, and voilà: a well-balanced diet with a variety of foods to meet nutritional needs and suit individual tastes.

Are there any foods which are just "empty calories"?

"Empty calories" is a term that has been bandied about for the last 10 to 15 years. It refers primarily to sugars, saturated fats, and alcohol because these three substances provide only calories without important nutrients such as protein, vitamins, or minerals. But *every* food we eat does not have to be chock full of nutrients, and as long as we eat a varied diet from the Basic Four, we will get plenty of all of the essential nutrients. The sugar, fat and alcohol can simply make meals taste better.

Most of the sugar we consume is consumed as a part of other foods. An example is ice cream, which is made essentially of whole milk, cream, and sugar. We like the taste largely because of the rich sweet taste, but when we eat ice cream we consume the nutrients found in milk. Another example is cake, which is usually made from flour, milk, eggs, fat, and sugar. Again, we eat the cake because of the pleasant rich, sweet taste, but we obtain the nutrients found in the wheat, milk, and eggs as well.

As Professor Edwin Bierman of the Department of Medicine, University of Washington, said: "There are no such things as 'empty' calories, only 'full' calories, full of energy."

What foods are "nutrient dense"?

The concept of nutrient density was developed by Dr. Garth Hanson while he was Professor of Nutrition at Utah State University, Logan.

"Nutrient dense" refers to the relative proportion of a specific nutrient to the amount of calories provided by the food. For example, skim milk has relatively few calories, yet has a high nutrient density in regard to calcium. Whole milk is generous in calories, has very little iron or ascorbic acid, and thus has low nutrient density in regard to these two nutrients. Yet, milk *is* a nutritious food, skim or whole. Thus, the use of this term is rather confusing (if not misleading). Butter is not considered to be a nutrient dense food, but it really is—in the nutrient fat!

A less confusing manner of evaluating the nutrient contributions of foods is by categorizing them individually into FOODS TO EMPHASIZE and FOODS TO DE-EMPHASIZE.

Foods to Emphasize

The practical dietary guidelines you may want to adhere to during the later years emphasize the inclusion of specific foodstuffs:

- **Protein foods** (around 15% total calories)
  Emphasis on low-fat choices such as vegetable protein combinations, skim/low-fat dairy products, fish, poultry, and lean meats.
- **Carbohydrate foods** (55 to 60% total calories)
  Emphasis on complex carbohydrates such as whole grain breads and cereals, dried beans and peas, pasta, potatoes and other starchy vegetables.
- **Vitamin heavy-weight foods** (C) Citrus fruits and their juices, Cantaloupe, Strawberries, Papaya, guava, mango, Cabbage, Cauliflower, Broccoli and other green leafy vegetables, Potatoes (with skins). (A) Liver, Apricots and other bright yellow fruits, Carrots, Tomato and other bright orange vegetables, Broccoli and other green leafy vegetables, Fortified low-fat milk, Fortified margarine, Fortified breakfast cereals. (D) Fortified milk, Fortified margarine, Fortified breakfast cereals, Fish liver oils, Liver. (B_1) Pork, lean cuts, Liver, Oysters, Whole grain and enriched breads and cereals, Dried beans and peas.
- **Mineral heavy-weight foods** (*Calcium*) Milk, skim or low-fat, Hard cheese, low-fat, Yogurt, low-fat, Oysters, Sardines and salmon (eaten with bones), Dark green leafy vegetables, Soybeans, fortified soy products. (*Iron*) Meat, especially organ meats (liver, kidneys, sweetbreads), Oysters, clams, Dried beans and peas, Whole grain and enriched breads and cereals, Dried fruits and their juices, Dark green leafy vegetables, Foods cooked in iron cookware.

Foods To De-Emphasize

Food can serve as one of life's greatest pleasures, and eating should be an enjoyable experience—at any age. Thus, it is undesirable to severely restrict your diet (unless your physician prescribes an individualized diet plan based on your personal health demands). Remember, following a flawless diet will not automatically grant you glowing health and immortality!

However, it is suggested that individuals of all ages should try to build a healthful diet to emphasize those foods which contain considerable quantities of vitamins, minerals, and/or fiber, but which are also caloric light-weights. Items which are sugar, fat, sodium and/or caloric heavy-weights should only be included in minimal amounts in your diet, and may need to be used with added caution as aging progresses:

Sugar heavy-weights—donuts, candy, flavored gelatin, cake, honey, jams, soft drinks, pastries, gum, ice cream, cookies, sugars, jellies, fruit-flavored drinks, presweetened cereals, sherbet, pie, syrups, preserves.
Fat heavy-weights—butter, fatty meats, bacon, chocolate, nuts, cream, fried foods, cream cheese, rich sweets, seeds, mayonnaise, gravies, sauces, sour cream, salad dressings, olives.
Sodium heavy-weights—bouillon, salted snack foods, luncheon meats, dried meats and fish, many condiments, soups, smoked or pickled items, bacon and ham, processed cheeses, certain seasonings.

Are the foods we need to de-emphasize considered "junk foods"?

No, not at all. Indeed, "junk foods" is a poor term, coined by pseudo-nutritionists who tend to belittle the American food industry. Those who use the term "junk food" usually refer to sweets, snackfoods, and many of the foods obtained in fast service restaurants such as hamburgers, hot dogs, french fries, pizza, etc. Yet, all foods can be part of a non-junky, healthful diet—but only a part. We still need to rely on fruits and vegetables, whole grain breads and cereals, milk and/or cheese, plus lean protein foods to have a well-balanced diet.

Actually, there are no such foods as "junk foods," since all foods when properly used in the diet contribute to health—both physiological and psychological. There are "junk diets"—those which are not varied and which are based on a few foods, whether fruits or burgers—but not "junk foods." As long as your diet is not leading to a problem of excess weight, sweets, snackfoods, and fast food fare can be included in moderate amounts.

If I do need to cut calories, what are the best items to minimize in my diet?

The "extra" foods, those you want to de-emphasize, are the first to go when minimizing caloric intake. Although such items are often favorites, high fat-calorie foods may be contributing to undesirable weight gain without enhancing either nutritional status or health. Therefore, if your calories need cutting, start with rich sweets such as cakes, donuts, pastries, pies, ice cream, and the like, skimp on fatty foods including butter and margarine, salad dressings, cream and sour cream, fried foods, and greasy choices, and cut back (or out) any alcoholic beverages. Some people find they need to eliminate in order to comply, but most people simply cut down rather than cut out, and can simultaneously cut calories without causing "diet depression" due to feelings of deprivation. For example, having the freedom to sip one cold "light" beer can wash away the chagrin which might plague any calorie-counting beer lover told to forgo his or her favorite brew!

How can I figure out the caloric contents of alcoholic beverages?

The alcoholic content of distilled spirits (gin, vodka, whiskey) is expressed in terms of "proof" which is equivalent to twice the alcohol content by volume. Thus, "100-proof" means 50 percent alcohol and "80-proof" is 40 percent alcohol. The alcohol in wine is expressed as a percentage, with table wines averaging 12–14% alcohol and the fortified wines (sherry, port) around 20–24%. Beers contain 3 to 5% alcohol, with light beers down toward the lower end of the spectrum and heavier ales at the opposite percent. A simple formula to determine the caloric content of an alcoholic beverage (without the mixer) is as follows: $0.8 \times \text{proof} \times \text{ounces} = \text{calories}$. Thus, the higher the proof, the more calories: but beer is usually guzzled by the 12-ounce can, wine sipped in 4-ounce glasses, alcohol served as 1-1/2 ounce shots plus mixer. The following charts illustrate caloric contents of popular alcoholic beverages and mixers:

Caloric Content of Alcoholic Beverages

Beverage	Proof	Amount (oz.)	Calories (Approx.)
Liquor, distilled	80	1½	95
	86	1½	105
	90	1½	115
	100	1½	125
Beer, "light"	3%	12	95
Beer, regular	4%	12	150
Ale	5	12	165
Wine, table	12	3½	90
Wine, fortified (sherry, port)	19	3½	140

Caloric Content of Mixers

Mixer, 6 ounces	Calories (Approx.)
Tonic	55
Collins	60
Ginger ale	60
Seven-Up	75
Cola	75
Fruit punch	80
Bitter lemon	85

Is alcohol unhealthy for the older person?

Usually not. In fact, in most cases a modest amount of alcohol helps one to relax, relieves stress and anxieties, and may frequently provide a little brighter outlook on life. But don't overdo a good thing, because too much will surely cause trouble.

Ruth Gordon

After chastising us on her questionnaire for failing to include a self-addressed, stamped envelope, Ruth Gordon immediately sent a follow-up apology in the "missing" envelope upon discovering that we had indeed provided her with one! As down-to-earth and filled with joie de vivre as her film characters portray, Ms. Gordon appears to drink in life: She is vibrantly alive and very active, but her diet is lean and her drinks are mean. Although the secret to long life may not lie in her daily Jack Daniels—one before dinner and two after—this ritual has not detracted from this still sparkling example of love of (long!) life. She is 88.

How much is a modest amount?

This varies with age and whether food is consumed with the alcoholic beverage. On empty stomachs, one drink is often more than enough. If consumed with a meal, or with generous quantities of hors d'oeuvres, then two should be the limit. One before bed may help you get to sleep, but none is plenty just before driving an automobile!

What about sugar—is it as "evil" as they say?

Sugar is certainly not evil, and most of us like the pleasant sweet taste of this much maligned foodstuff. As with everything else, it is best not to overdo on sugar. Yet it is not necessary to restrict intake out of unnecessary fears. Except for implications in dental decay, *sugar has never been shown to cause any ills in humans.* Despite scare tactics to the contrary, moderate sugar consumption does not lead to heart disease, cancer, obesity, diabetes, arthritis, nor to fatigue, behavioral disorders, mental illness, crime, baldness, blindness or any other disorder, vague or serious. And in oral decay, it is more important to consider the frequency of sugar consumption and what form it is eaten in, rather than the amount. If one eats sugar a number of times during the day, and in sticky forms which adhere to the teeth, the decay activity of carbohydrates is prolonged. If sugar is eaten less frequently as part of meals (followed by toothbrushing/flossing) and in less sticky form, there is less decay production, no matter what amount of sugar is consumed.

As far as sugar consumption in this country is concerned, we tend to use about 130 lbs (including corn sweeteners) per year. However, since a sizable amount of this "food disappearance" figure is wasted—sugar crumbs falling off sweets, sugar left in the bottom of the coffee cup, sugar used in fermenting foods, etc.—the total amount actually eaten is less.

You need not avoid sugar due to false beliefs in inherent dangers, and may find that an occasional treat is a luxury you want to be able to afford yourself. After all, food is meant to provide pleasure as well as nutrition.

Milton Berle

Milton Berle may make us laugh, but he takes his diet—and his health—seriously. Once less aware of his eating habits than he is today, "Uncle Milty" currently uses care in planning his daily menus: He limits the intake of red meats in favor of chicken or fish, restricts salt, alcohol and caffeine, and rarely eats fried foods; breakfast includes whole grain toast, lunch is usually a healthful salad, and dinner a well-balanced meal including entrée, vegetable, rice or potatoes, salad and dessert—on occasion, his "weakness—chocolate cake"! Regular physical activity in the form of walking and golf helps to keep Milton Berle looking trim—despite his choco-indulgences!

Is honey a more nutritious choice?

No, honey is not more nutritious than ordinary sugar from the sugar bowl. True, honey has a speck of nutrients—a few vitamins and minerals—but not in any significant amounts. For example, if you wanted to obtain the same amount of calcium from honey as you can get in a glass of milk, you would have to consume almost 300 tablespoons! This means about 18,000 calories, compared to less than 100 in a glass of low-fat milk. This is true of the other nutrients present in honey: the amounts are quite insignificant.

Honey has a different taste, and for good noses, some have pleasant aromas which vary from honey to honey. If you like the taste of honey, use it occasionally in place of sugar. But in so doing, don't swallow the stories of superior nutritional qualities you may also be receiving, because these are nil. Although honey is sweeter than sugar, it is doubtful that you will reduce your caloric intake much by substituting honey for table sugar. *Note:* Honey can also have health implications not bargained for, because it has been linked to botulism poisoning in infants, and some of the "natural" *un*refined types have caused other ills in adults.

What about using saccharin and aspartame instead of sugar?

Saccharin and aspartame, the newer low-calorie sweeteners, are OK if you find them psychologically pleasing, but they will probably not prove helpful in weight reduction. In fact, there has yet to appear a single paper in the scientific or medical literature indicating that either sweetener is really helpful in weight reduction efforts! Both of these sweeteners are safe to use, although some individuals (usually young children or those with an inherited disease called PKU or phenyl-ketonuria) should not use foods or beverages to which aspartame has been added. Read the label: it will warn you of any problems of intake of which you need to be aware.

So if sugar isn't the culprit and a small quantity of alcoholic beverages is OK, what is the dietary villain we need to watch out for?

You have two *dietary* villains to look out for: eating too much in relation to your physical activities so that you put on too many undesired pounds, and eating meals that have little variety and are not selected from the Basic Four Food Groups. With too little variety, there is a good chance of not getting adequate amounts of the 50 or so nutrients needed over the long haul for the best nutrition. The worst villain, however, is the one scaring you about the many delicious and nutritious foods available for you to enjoy, not fear.

FOOD FADDISM—CONSUMER BEWARE!

Is there really no need for older individuals to take food supplements?

This is seldom necessary for individuals—at any age—who are eating a well-balanced, varied diet and who are in reasonably good health, particularly if they have no diseases of the intestinal tract or other disorders which interfere with the absorption or utilization of nutrients. Unless prescribed by a physician based on an individualized diagnosis, food supplements—protein powders, bottles of non-nutrients and special elixirs, "life extension" formulas, etc.—are simply additions to the long rows on "health food" store shelves of unnecessary, expensive, and sometimes dangerous potions, hyped up by pseudo-nutritionists hoping to make money from naive consumers.

Which herbs can cause undesirable side effects?

Just because something is "natural" does not guarantee its safety—ask any well-seasoned mushroom hunter about that concept. Herbs have long been touted for medicinal properties, from folklore to "health food" store, yet many are actually dangerous to your health. Some even have fatal results for unwary users.

Adverse Effects of Herbs

Herb	Adverse Effects
Chamomile (camomile), goldenrod, marigold, yarrow	Allergic reactions, including fatal allergic shock in persons sensitive to ragweed, asters, chrysanthemums and related plants
Poke root	Nausea, vomiting, cramps, diarrhea
Buchu, quack grass, dandelion	Diuresis (loss of body water)
Catnip, juniper, hydrangea, jimson weed, lobelia, nutmeg, wormwood	Nervous system damage, hallucinations
Burdock root	Atropine-like symptoms (blurred vision, dry mouth, hallucinations)
Buckthorn bark, dock root, aloe leaves	Diarrhea
Senna (leaves, flowers, bark)	Cramps, diarrhea
Sassafras root bark	A carcinogen (cancer-causing agent)
St. John's wort	Delayed allergic reactions, sun sensitivity
Pennyroyal, Indian tobacco, shavegrass (horsetail), mistletoe leaves	Death
Ginseng, licorice	Elevated blood pressure
Comfrey	Liver damage

Are there any other dangerous "health foods"?

The list is quite extensive for those items promoted to increase health which actually can detract from well-being, even to the point of being life-threatening. The following table* may give you a general idea of those items you would be wise to avoid in your next trip to a local "health food" store or "natural" restaurant—there are plenty of others, however, and new items are appearing every day for which "caveat emptor" (buyer beware) may apply:

Alfalfa—Although advocates of this plant suggest that it offers certain nutrients that other more common plant foods do not, alfalfa actually has less nutritional value than most of the more popular vegetables such as broccoli, carrots and spinach. Claims have also been made that alfalfa contains all of the essential amino acids, but this is untrue. Fans of alfalfa supplements and extracts promise the additional benefits of "anti-toxin properties" and the ability to "prevent exhaustion." There is no scientific evidence to support these claims. Alfalfa tea, one of the currently popular herbal teas, contains saponins which can adversely affect digestion and respiration.

Aloe vera—Despite the various claims made by proponents of this plant, aloe juice has never been shown to be an effective cure for arthritis or any other health problem. Using aloe creams and gels on your skin is probably harmless, and even though it won't reverse the inevitable process of aging, topical aloe may exert some skin-softening and

*Table adapted from Stare and Aronson's *Your Basic Guide to Nutrition* (George F. Stickley Co., 1983).

moisturizing effects. However, ingested aloe juice acts as a laxative and can cause gastrointestinal upset.

If you like rubbing aloe-containing creams onto your skin, by all means do so. But you should steer clear of using aloe as a food supplement, oral medicine or menu item. Internally, the aloe plant is useless at best, and can even be dangerous.

Bone meal—Powdered bone is sold through "health food" stores and advertised in magazines as a rich source of calcium. Actually, calcium from this source is poorly absorbed. More significantly, many bone meal samples have been found to contain high levels of lead (a toxic mineral). Thus, bone meal supplements are useless and can be dangerous.

Bran—As one of the fibers of wheat grain, bran is composed mainly of cellulose. It is effective against constipation, but so are whole grains and generous amounts of fruits and vegetables in the diet. However, the claim that bran can lower cholesterol is untrue. Excessive intake of bran can lead to loss of minerals and gastrointestinal disturbances.

Chelated minerals—"Chelate" simply means "to bind." Minerals in chelated supplements are usually bound to protein in order to enhance their absorption into the body. Mineral supplements should never be taken unless prescribed by a physician. Individuals with a *medically diagnosed* need for mineral supplements can get adequate amounts from non-chelated forms, which are less expensive.

Dolomite—Dolomite, mined from rocks, contains calcium and magnesium. However, these minerals are poorly absorbed from dolomite supplements and are often accompanied by large amounts of toxic metals. Lead, arsenic, mercury and other contaminants have been found in dolomite samples in amounts ample enough to damage health. Obviously, milk and milk products are more sensible sources of calcium; and legumes, green leafy vegetables and whole grains can more safely supply the magnesium we need.

Ginseng—Ginseng is one of the more popular plants used for making herbal teas. Used in the occult world for centuries, ginseng derives its name from the Chinese words for "man-plant" because the root often looks as if it has arms and legs. Ginseng is now promoted as a cure-all for illnesses ranging from impotence and stress to heart disease and cancer. It has been touted as an ancient potion bearing "magical" powers, and is marketed to those who are seeking an edible fountain of youth which guarantees good health and long life. Claims are also made that use of this herb can provide a "joyful temper, plenty of pure red blood, relief for your irritable bladder," and increased sexual pleasure.

Unfortunately for naive consumers, ginseng has never been shown to provide any health benefits. In fact, the overuse of ginseng can produce a variety of problems including elevated blood pressure, a particularly dangerous side effect in individuals with hypertension. Other side effects include nervousness, insomnia, confusion, depression and gastrointestinal disorders.

GTF chromium—GTF (glucose tolerance factor) chromium is derived from yeast that has been grown in a chromium-rich medium, or can be isolated from pork kidney. Health claims associated with this product include increases in energy and stamina, improvements in cardiovascular fitness, and a strengthened sense of overall well-being. Although chromium is known to be an essential nutrient, a varied diet provides an adequate supply. Glowing claims for GTF chromium supplements are highly exaggerated.

Kelp—Kelp is a seaweed common in the Japanese diet. Tablets of kelp are prepared from dried seaweed and promoted in "health food" stores as a weight reduction aid, rich source of the mineral iodide, an energy booster, and a "natural" cure for certain ailments including goiter. True, kelp is high in iodide, and a deficiency of this mineral can lead to goiter. But iodized salt contributes plenty of this mineral to our diets, and at a fraction of the cost. Excess iodide can be detrimental to your health and can also lead to the development of goiter.

Kelp is high in sodium, a mineral we tend to overconsume anyway, but it is not a significant source of calories (hence energy), nor of any other nutrients—aside from the two minerals mentioned—that are required by the body. The urine of some individuals taking kelp tablets has been found to contain elevated levels of arsenic, a poison which may possibly be carcinogenic as well. "Natural" foods are not always health-promoting, and nutritional supplements often cause more problems than their proponents talk about.

Laetrile—Laetrile is sometimes referred to as "vitamin B_{17}," but there is actually no such vitamin—and laetrile is certainly not a vitamin! Laetrile is the chemical, amygdalin, which is found naturally in the pits of peaches, apricots, bitter almonds, and some other plant materials. There is no scientific evidence that laetrile inhibits the development or growth of cancer cells.

The so-called "evidence" presented by laetrile supporters has consisted of testimonials given by various individuals who believe that laetrile has cured them of cancer. One well-known advocate of laetrile was asked to submit files of his most dramatic cases of success to the Food and Drug Administration. Of the nine records reviewed, six patients had died of cancer, one still had cancer—which had spread since laetrile had been taken—one had used approved drugs and radiation therapy, and one had died of another disease after having had the cancer surgically removed.

Laetrile is not harmless. It contains significant amounts of one of the most toxic substances known: cyanide. More important, many people have died as a result of taking laetrile in place of proper medical treatment for cancer. The modern health quack has learned to reach people emotionally. It is certainly not very difficult to sell hope to people who are desperate.

Protein supplements—Protein powders, tablets and liquids have been advertised as strength-promoting and especially important to athletes. These claims are incorrect. It is quite easy to obtain all the protein your body requires through a well-balanced dietary intake. Meat, poultry, fish, eggs, milk and cheese (as well as certain plant food combinations) provide plenty of the protein essential for good health. Nor do athletes require extra protein. As a sole food source, or in excessive amounts, protein supplements can cause nutritional imbalances, kidney problems, and ill health.

Raw milk—Pasteurization is one of the important technological advances that have led to improved standards of health and safety for today's consumers. The ungrounded fear that pasteurization destroys some important nutrients in milk has caused some naive consumers to endanger their health by consuming "certified" milk or other types of raw (unpasteurized) milk. Although about 10 percent of the heat-sensitive vitamins (vitamin C, B_{12}, thiamin) are destroyed in the pasteurizing process, milk is not a significant source of these nutrients. On the other hand, contaminated raw milk can be a source of harmful bacteria, such as those which cause undulant fever, dysentery, and tuberculosis. ("Certified" means that the cows have been tested free of tuberculosis, but it does not mean that the milk can't contain other disease-producing organisms.) Why expose yourself to a serious disease when there is nothing to gain in return?

"*Vitamin* B_{15}"—Like B_{17}, the substance labeled B_{15} is not a vitamin. Also known as pangamate, pangamic acid, or "Russian Formula," this product has now become one of the most popular nutrition supplements, despite the lack of evidence to support its use for any health reason.

"Pangamate is a label, not a substance," says Dr. Victor Herbert, Chairman of the Department of Medicine at Hahnemann University in Philadelphia. It appears that sellers toss any chemicals they choose into bottles and label them "Vitamin B_{15}" or "pangamate," so that consumers have no way of knowing exactly what they are purchasing.

B_{15} can be hazardous because the chemicals typically present in the supplements often have dangerous side effects. Manufacturers frequently make B_{15} with a chemical known as DIPA, which causes blood pressure to drop, and this results in the "kick" users believe to be due to "vitamin power." Actually, DIPA is a poison and is believed to be cancer-causing. Another chemical sold as B_{15} is N,N-dimethylglycine hydrochloride (DMG), a substance Dr. Herbert believes may cause cancer.

The many claims made for vitamin B_{15} include the treatment of cancer, heart disease, alcoholism, diabetes, glaucoma, allergies and schizophrenia. Supposedly, it can purify the air, provide the body with instant oxygen, and slow down the aging process. Yet there exists absolutely no proof that B_{15} has any therapeutic benefit, or even that it is safe to ingest. B_{15} is another example of a phony nutrient which is helpful only to those who sell it.

The Food and Drug Administration considers "vitamin B_{15}" to be a food additive for which no evidence of safety has been offered. It is therefore illegal for the substance to be sold as a dietary supplement.

What *are* "health foods," if they do not supply health benefits?

"Health foods" are usually healthy only in their prices, and are more often than not advertising rip-offs. In fact, the term is as meaningless as "junk foods" in that all foods are health foods when properly included in the diet, as a varied diet contributes to good health, both physical and psychological. No one food is especially health-promoting, but a diet can be quite healthful if based on a variety of nutritious foods. An apple a day may not keep the doctor away, but a varied diet which may include apples—as well as many other fruits, vegetables, grains, milk products, meats and alternates—can help to keep illnesses at bay.

Your local "health food" store may only sell products which are no more healthy for you than similar foods bought in any supermarket or grocery store, yet are priced considerably higher. A 1983 report by the New York City Department of Consumer Affairs concluded: "Consumers will do little to aid their health by shopping at overpriced health food stores. They may even harm it." The report also stated that "health foods do not differ significantly from conventional foods in terms of nutritional value, pesticide residue level, appearance, and taste. The major difference the Department found between health foods and conventional foods is the much higher cost of the former."

"Health food" stores base a large part of their business on the many brands of food supplements—vitamins and minerals, protein powders, added fibers, fructose and sweeteners, non-nutrients, etc.—which are usually not even necessary to ingest, and tend to be higher priced than comparable supplements in pharmacies or even department stores. But why not get your nutrients—all that you need—from your local supermarket in a more natural form (i.e., a variety of nutritious and delicious foods) and at a far lower price?

Then are the so-called "natural" foods any more healthful than other products?

Another meaningless term, like "junk" and "health" when applied to food, "natural" has no legal or clearly accepted definition. This label once was restricted to items touted in "health food" stores, but was adopted by the food industry and applied to everything from cereals and cheeses to beer and chips. Due to the public's naive preference for "natural" (versus synthetic or industry-produced) products, everything from shampoo to pet food carries this misleading label. Most "natural" products cost more than their "unnatural" equivalents. Why pay more—unless, of course, you favor the brand or some of the possible benefits the product may provide (e.g., low-sodium, low-calorie, low-fat, unsweetened, no caffeine, etc.) to meet your individual needs or desires—for the so-called "natural" products which simply *cost* you more without *giving* you anything at all. Read the label—beyond the enticing and bold "All Natural" tag.

Do "organic" foods supply more nutrients in a less contaminated form than other products?

Again, a term seized on by advertisers to promote products at increased costs without added benefits for unknowing consumers: "organic" means only that the product contains carbon, which is true for all foods. In today's market places, however, an "organic" label denotes a higher price. Many consumers believe that they are purchasing products without preservatives, additives, or pesticide residues, but this is not always the case with "organic" foods. Several studies found that items labeled "organic" contained *more* pesticide residue than their supermarket counterparts! This may be due to water or air-borne pesticide residues which "contaminate" the "organic" produce, or to produce salespersons who try to take advantage of unwary purchasers. In either case, the consumer loses out by spending more money for similar supermarket fare.

Also, pesticides—as well as additives and preservatives—are not "contaminants," but chemicals used in minute quantities to provide us with a varied and nutrient-rich food supply. Without these chemicals, our foods would wilt and deteriorate before ever reaching our kitchens, or would have shelf-lives of limited lengths: No oranges in the Northeast, no seafood in the Midwest, and head for South America for a good cup of coffee; stale breads, insect-ridden cereals, and ruined crop after ruined crop would be normal daily news for the "au natural" consumer. Besides, there is nothing wrong with chemicals—all foods are composed of chemicals, even your body is made up of chemicals. Our food supply is the safest, most varied, and most nutritious in all of history—with many thanks to our invisible friends, the chemicals.

Does this mean that older people can obtain all of the nutrients they need simply by following a well-balanced diet based on a variety of foods from the Basic Four Food Groups and purchased in the local supermarket?

Yes! This is the key to a well-balanced and enjoyable diet at prices you can afford: variety, moderation, and taste combine your favorite foods into menu plans which suit your nutritional needs and individual tastes. No need to rely on expensive supplements, special foods labeled as "health" or "natural" or "organic" nor to restrict your diet under the misconception that "chemicals" and "junk foods" are to be avoided. Instead, you can easily build a practical diet plan around the Basic Four Food Groups, one that you can afford to purchase, are able to prepare, and may certainly enjoy—physically and psychologically. This goes for your children, grandchildren and any other generations waiting in the wings!

Now that I'm "golden," just how do I learn to adhere to a perfect diet?

As you grow older, the various fluctuations which may occur in your lifestyle patterns are reflected in eating habits, dietary constructions, and levels of physical activity. Therefore, it is impractical to hold unrealistic expectations regarding your own capabilities for lifelong adherence to a flawless lifestyle. In this current age of fast-paced living patterns with their major daily changes, strict adherence to a model diet and exercise pattern is improbable, if not impossible. And leading a "perfect" lifestyle could most certainly prove to be boring!

Even when you're "golden," your diet need not be dull in order to be healthful. Yet it is important for you to realize the enormous influence of diet and exercise on the aging body. Excessive gain or loss of weight, erratic eating habits and unbalanced meals, alcohol abuse, and sedentary living patterns do not contribute to a strong foundation for prolonged health. If you burden your heart and blood vessels with a fat, inactive body and fat-laden diet, you may enter the later stages of life in a prematurely aged condition. Inadequate nutrition can cause deficiency diseases and the undesirable side effects such as loss of teeth, fragile bones, anemias, susceptibility to infection, and other ailments. Prolonged malnutrition, or the "overnutrition" which leads to obesity, might even snuff out your life just short of the "golden years." So, although it is unnecessary and impractical to seek out the "perfect" diet, it is important to optimize your diet for a healthy, happy, "golden" lifetime. This simply means:

1) Follow a well-balanced diet which includes a variety of foods in moderate amounts.
2) Select your foods from the Basic Four Food Groups—and be sure to have some of your favorites—in portions which help you to maintain a reasonable weight.
3) Emphasize fruits, vegetables, breads and cereals, plus low-fat dairy foods and lean meats, while you de-emphasize high-fat foods, rich sweets, and alcoholic beverages—but remember: There's no need to deprive yourself to the point of "dietary depression"!
4) Watch out for food fads, magical diets, superfoods, health "cures," and other tempting but misleading dietary sales pitches: Save your money and your health by being an alert consumer.

Part II

First Course: Getting in Shape, Sensibly

FIRST COURSE: GETTING IN SHAPE, SENSIBLY

How is your self-image these days? Do you consider yourself to be "in shape," or just "as good as can be expected at your age"? With a gradual decline in your level of activity—a common trend as one grows older—you may have noticed one of two bodily changes: loss of an appetite for food, with loss of weight; or, undesired weight gain–a little bit at a time, it has gradually added up.

If the former weight problem is affecting your self-image, it will also detract from your overall health, damaging your emotional and even physical well-being. Although a less common complaint these days for Americans of all ages, underweight can pose a puzzling dietary problem: how to gain pounds to attain a reasonable weight without force-feeding. The following tips may assist those in the often envied need-to-gain-a-few group (for those who become extremely under-weight with age—that is, more than 20% below the norms for age/sex/height—consultation with a physician should be obtained to rule out any possible underlying disease):

- Eat smaller meals, but eat more often. Try to build a regular meal/ snack pattern into your daily schedule so that you don't forget to eat. If you keep portion sizes small, food may not appear to be so overwhelming.
- Stimulate your appetite by making meals with appeal. Vary the flavors, textures, temperatures of the food, and vary your eating environment. Fix up an attractive meal tray, sit out on the porch, and invite a guest to join you, for example.
- Fortify your foods to sneak in those extra calories. Make shakes with non-fat dried milk and a few scoops of ice cream. Scoop some more non-fat dried milk into other foods such as meatloaf, doughs and batters, or puddings. Cheese-up your casseroles, soups, sand-wiches.
- Spread the peanut butter THICK . . . on toast, raw vegetable sticks, muffins, and quick breads. And don't be afraid to experi-ment. Try it, you'll like it!

Older women tend to have inadequate caloric intakes more often than their male counterparts, but in either sex—as at any age—meager meals means suboptimal nutrition. This can easily lead to poor health. If you've found yourself dwindling with the years and sliding too far down on the thin scale, spark up your diet and watch your health—and your self-image—begin to glow.

The bulk of those in their later years, however, are contesting with the opposite and equally puzzling dietary problem: how to lose pounds to attain a reasonable weight without starving, suffering from "diet depression," and ruining both physical and emotional health. As you have grown older, you may have found that the battle of the bulges has become more and more of a struggle. Fortunately, with the adoption of proper lifestyle patterns, the diet war can be transformed into a stimulating challenge. You may soon find that this challenge is one you really enjoy tackling every day, no matter how old you are, and will continue to enjoy doing—for a lifetime. Meeting the daily lifestyle demands head on with a smile—and eventually in a healthy, trim, youthful body—can do wonders for your self-image.

Participating in the next two chapters can help you to alter your lifestyle to improve your diet and exercise patterns. By following a sensible diet and adopting a daily exercise plan, you can add life to your years, if not years to your life. Go for it!

It seems like I gain several more pounds of undesired fat every year, and I'm not eating any more than I used to. Does aging cause weight gain?

As your body ages, a process which begins at birth and continues throughout your lifetime, there are continual changes in your physical (and emotional!) structure. With growth during infancy, childhood, and the teenage years, your body needs more energy (calories) for building new tissues. This is also true during pregnancy, and for those women who breastfeed and thus require calories for milk production.

However, once you reach your 20's, the body stops growing and begins to slow down in the overall rate of functioning: by the time you reach age 65, the rate at which your body functions ("metabolism") may be 12% to 20% lower than it was at age 20. This is largely because body composition changes with aging, with a shift away from metabolically active body lean (muscle tissue) towards deposition of more of the less-calorie-burning body fat. The chart below illustrates the typical body make-up changes which account for much of the age-related decline in caloric needs.

It is interesting to note that researchers are still not sure whether it is the aging process itself which causes these physical alterations, or if it is a decrease in physical activity. With regular exercise, the age-related accumulation of fat can be arrested—or at least minimized. More on physical activity later.

Since your body's metabolism has slowed, you will need to curtail your caloric intake to compensate for the reduced energy need. However, your nutrient needs have not similarly decreased, so you should avoid the elimination of nutrient-rich foods from your diet. This means that older folks have to be especially careful to select a variety of

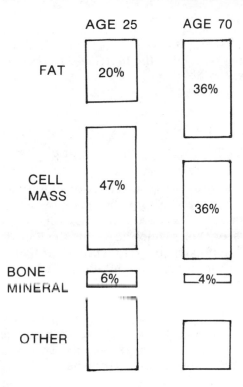

Body composition and age of men: Body fat increases, while cell mass and bone mineral decrease as age progresses after maturity. (From Gregerman, R.I. and Bierman, E.I., *Textbook of Endocrinology*, R.H. Williams, ed. Philadelphia, W.B. Saunders Co. 1974.)

nutritious foods at each meal and snack. Fortunately we tend to grow wiser with age, and that can mean nutritionally more knowledgeable, too!

If food is so important to older people, then how can we drop the unwanted pounds?

The best method to improve your weight status is by adopting a safe, effective, sensible diet plan—one you can live with. We call this lifestyle pattern the "Four-Prong Approach to Weight Control":

1) Well-balanced diet at caloric level to reach and maintain reasonable weight;
2) Regular program of physical exercise to use up calories, speed up body metabolism, and lift up spirits and self-image;

3) Behavioral changes to establish lifestyle patterns conducive to optimal well-being; and

4) Attitude-shaping so that the motivation to become and stay fit is permanently established.

THE FOUR-PRONG APPROACH

Most weight loss programs focus only on dietary intake, some may encourage exercise, a few also incorporate behavioral modification plans. Unfortunately, there are very few—if any—weight control books, programs, or clinics which advocate the Four-Prong Approach. Yet, with the information required to establish an individualized weight control plan, you can utilize the Four-Prong Approach on your own: The first chapter of this book outlined the basics of nutrition, which can be incorporated into a sensible weight loss plan as described in this chapter; the next chapter explains how to embark on a specific exercise program; the behavioral changes appropriate for becoming fit are provided in all of the chapters, as are tips on reshaping a sagging attitude into the motivation required for a new fit-for-life you. Read on!

The Well-Balanced Diet

Can you outline a sensible weight loss diet?

The three plans outlined below allow you to choose the foods you want to eat at each meal and snack in order to follow a 1000-, 1200- or 1500-calorie diet. Read through these plans carefully and select the calorie level which will allow you to lose weight without going hungry. For inactive females, the 1000-calorie plan may be best—but get active, too, if possible—whereas more active females and males may find that the 1500-calorie plan is suitable. If you find that you are losing weight too rapidly, more than 1 to 2 pounds per week, switch to a higher calorie diet. If you are not losing weight as you desire, perhaps you need to try a plan allowing less calories—and/or increase your exercise level. The diet plans are given on the pages following, each with allowed daily food group servings, meal pattern, plus a sample menu to illustrate how to make food selections within the plan. Serving sizes for each of the Basic Four Food Groups are also given, plus serving sizes of "fats" and "luxury" foods. Note that one asterisk (*) indicates that the food contains fat equivalent to 1/2-fat serving; when eating (*) foods, eliminate 1/2-fat serving from your total allowed daily food group servings. Two asterisk foods (**) contain fat equivalent to one fat serving; when eating (**) foods, eliminate one fat serving from your total allowed daily food group servings. (Does this seem confusing? It may be somewhat difficult to understand at first, but will soon prove to be an easy, fast method to keep track of your fat intake.)

You may want to post your diet plan and serving sizes on your refrigerator or kitchen cupboard for easy access during menu planning.

So, start now! You are on your way to optimal health through improved nutrition.

1000 DIET PLAN
(1000 calories)

Allowed Daily Food Group Servings:

Fruit-2   Milk and Cheese-2   Vegetable-2
Meat and Alternates-4   Grain-4   Fat-3
+Luxury

Meal Pattern	Sample Menu (with serving equivalents)
Breakfast	
1 Grain	1/2 cup oatmeal (1 Grain)
1/2 Milk	1/2 cup skim milk (1/2 Milk)
1 Fruit	2 tbsp raisins (1 Fruit)
	coffee, black (unlimited)
Lunch	Sandwich:
1 Meat	1/4 cup tuna fish (1 Meat)
1 Fat	2 tsp low-calorie mayonnaise (1 Fat)
1 Grain	2 sl thin-slice wheat bread (1 Grain)
	lettuce (unlimited)
1 Milk	1 cup skim milk (1 Milk)
1 Fruit	1 tangerine
Supper	
3 Meat	3 oz broiled chicken (3 Meat)
1 Grain	1 small baked potato (1 Grain)
2 Fat	2 tbsp sour cream (1 Fat)
2 Veg	1/2 cup asparagus, steamed (1 Veg)
	tossed salad:
	lettuce (unlimited)
	1/2 cup mixed raw veg (1 Veg)
	low-calorie dressing (1 Fat)
Luxury	1 av slice sponge cake (Luxury)
Snacks	
1 Grain	3 whole rye crackers (1 Grain)
1/2 Milk	1/2 cup skim milk (1/2 Milk)

1200 DIET PLAN
(1200 Calories)

Allowed Daily Food Group Servings:

Fruit-4   Milk and Cheese-2   Vegetable-2
Meat and Alternates-5   Grain-5   Fat-3
+Luxury

Meal Pattern	Sample Menu (with serving equivalents)
Breakfast	
1 Grain	1 cup puffed rice cereal (1 Grain)
1/2 Milk	1/2 cup skim milk (1/2 Milk)
1 Fruit	1/2 sm banana (1 Fruit)
	coffee, black (unlimited)
Lunch	Sandwich:
1 Meat	1 oz diced chicken (1 Meat)
1 Fat	2 tsp low-calorie mayonnaise (1 Fat)
2 Grain	2 sl oatmeal bread (2 Grain)
	lettuce (unlimited)
1 Milk	1 cup skim milk (1 Milk)
1 Fruit	1 sm orange (1 Fruit)
Supper	
4 Meat	4 oz veal (4 Meat) broiled with
2 Veg	1/2 cup mushrooms (1 Veg) in
2 Fat	1 tsp vegetable oil (1 Fat)
	tossed salad:
	lettuce (unlimited)
	1/2 cup mixed raw veg (1 Veg)
	low-calorie dressing (1 Fat)
1 Grain	1/2 cup brown rice (1 Grain)
1 Fruit	1/4 small cantaloupe (1 Fruit)
Luxury	5 gingersnaps (Luxury)
Snacks	
1 Grain	3 cups popcorn (1 Grain)
1 Fruit	Slim Shake:
	1/2 cup strawberries (1 Fruit)
1/2 Milk	1/2 cup skim milk (1/2 Milk)
	crushed ice (unlimited)

James Beard

One might expect that this well-known gourmet cook might also be a gourmand, but James Beard's current diet is reflective of his belief in sensible eating and moderation in all things. Once a hefty eater who also very much enjoyed his mealtime wines and alcoholic beverages, Beard has altered his dietary patterns (under a physician's guidance) to emphasize plain-'n-simple fare: plenty

1500 DIET PLAN
(1500 Calories)

Allowed Daily Food Group Servings:

Fruit-6   Milk and Cheese-2   Vegetable-2
Meat and Alternates-6   Grain-6   Fat-5
+ Luxury

Meal Pattern	Sample Menu (with serving equivalents)
Breakfast	
1 Grain	3/4 cup shredded wheat cereal (1 Grain)
1/2 Milk	1/2 cup skim milk (1/2 Milk)
2 Fruit	1/2 banana (1 Fruit)
	1/2 cup orange juice (1 Fruit)
	coffee, black (unlimited)
Lunch	Sandwich:
2 Meat	2 oz boiled ham (2 Meat + 1 Fat)
? Fat	1-1/2 oz part skim mozzarella cheese
1 Milk	(1 Milk + 1 Fat)
	mustard (unlimited)
2 Grain	2 sl whole rye bread (2 Grain)
	lettuce (unlimited)
2 Fruit	1 fresh pear (2 Fruit)
Supper	
4 Meat	4 oz (1 oz each) lean meatballs (4 Meat + 2 Fat)
3 Fat	1/2 cup tomato sauce (1 Veg + 1 Fat)
2 Veg	
2 Grain	1 cup whole wheat spaghetti (2 Grain)
	Italian salad:
	lettuce (unlimited)
	1/4 cup sliced tomatoes (1/2 Veg)
	1/4 cup cold green beans (1/2 Veg)
	Lemon and vinegar (unlimited)
1 Fruit	10 to 12 fresh cherries (1 Fruit)
Luxury	1 av slice angel food cake (Luxury)
Snacks	
1 Grain	1/2 whole wheat English muffin (1 Grain) with
1 Fruit	1/2 apple, sliced (1 Fruit) sprinkled with
	cinnamon (unltd.)
1/2 Milk	1/2 cup skim milk (1/2 Milk)

of fresh fruits, vegetables, breads and salads have replaced the less lean cuisine of old. Even those who know food best—that is, the gourmet cooks, nutrition professionals, and long-lived food lovers—opt for sensible eating in order to enable themselves to enjoy food healthfully, longer! and James Beard did; he died recently at the age of 81.

The diet makes sense, but the calories are confusing. What exactly is a calorie?

Calories are not nutrients, but a unit measure of energy: With foods, calories refer to the energy obtained by the body when the foods are digested, absorbed and metabolized; with exercise or physical activity, calories refer to the energy required (used up) in conducting the exercise or activity. Physicists define a calorie as the amount of energy required to raise the temperature of 1 milliliter of water (about 1/5 of a teaspoonful) 1 degree centigrade. The nutritionist and physiologist define a calorie as a thousand times more than the physical (i.e., to raise the temperature of 1000 milliliters of water—a little more than a quart—1 degree centigrade). This is correctly referred to as a *kilocalorie* or by spelling calorie with a capital C (Calorie). But since it is impractical to measure in calories (e.g., 1 apple would have 60,000 calories versus 60 kilocalories), and because it is a mouthful to use the term *kilocalories*, we measure in kilocalories but talk in calories.

Remember that the energy-nutrients are protein and carbohydrate (with 4 calories per gram each) and fat (9 calories per gram); alcohol also provides non-nutritious calories (7 per gram). The other nutrients—vitamins, minerals, and water—as well as fiber do not provide the body with energy, hence, are non-caloric.

It is important to understand that calorie charts are not very accurate reflections of the energy values of the foods you eat. Instead, these charts are guides to assist you in estimating caloric intake. For example, an apple may be listed in a calorie chart as providing 60 calories—but is it a big or small apple, sweet or tart, do you eat it core and all or just nibble on well-pared slices? Obviously, caloric estimates are objective and variable, so don't think that a slice of cake the size of your head totals 250 calories as listed for an "average portion." Calorie charts can help you to determine your average intakes, but the numbers can easily be used to your disadvantage as well.

Sensible Dieting Vs. Fads or Phonies

Why is it wise to follow a 1000 or 1200-calorie diet in attempting to lose weight? Why not cut calorie intake real low and shed the pounds faster?

With a daily caloric intake of 1000–1200 calories, and a modest increase in physical activity, one will lose weight gradually at an average of one to two pounds per week or 4 to 8 pounds per month. Such a gradual weight loss is much more likely to be retained for a period of months or even years than if one drastically reduces caloric intake and quickly sheds the excess poundage. Chances are good that you did not put on all those extra pounds in just a few weeks, but over a period of years. Therefore, you cannot expect to take the pounds off in a short period of only a few weeks—or overnight!

Although "crash" diets are popular—first one type then another new plan is the rage, you will probably find that only your hopes crash— none of these diets works permanently. A rapid weight loss is usually due to loss of body fluids, not fat, which reaccumulate just as rapidly once the crash dieter resumes normal eating patterns. Body fat is not lost, and the unfortunate dieter tends to rebound after the diet with a gain of more fat. If a crash diet *did* work, it would be here to stay—not a fad, as they all are.

Such fad diets are nutritionally unbalanced and, although usually only followed for short periods of time, such diets can threaten nutritional status. These diets tend to be low in carbohydrate, sometimes protein, usually iron and calcium, as well as other minerals and various vitamins. Overall, the crash diets are as barren nutritionally as they are psychologically: lose weight by robbing your body of nutrients and your psyche of eating enjoyment—bore your weight off!

There are a number of health hazards associated with "crash" diets, in addition to the nutritional imbalance. A rapid loss of weight and a low caloric intake usually leaves one rather weak and tired and can cause a number of health problems such as low blood pressure, headache, dizziness, nausea, electrolyte imbalance, ketosis (metabolic imbalance), plus coma, heart irregularities, and even death! By drastically altering your lifestyle to follow some temporary diet craze, you do nothing to change the habits which have led to the undesired weight gain. Thus, crash diets do not improve your dietary behavior to ward off weight *regain*. Weight is almost always (over 90% of the time) regained, usually rather rapidly. Certainly not the intelligent way to reach and maintain a reasonable weight, "crash" diets are best left to those who unwisely elect to be on a rollercoaster ride with weight control.

But to get started on my weight loss program, wouldn't it help to fast first, or go on some other quick-shrink scheme just to get me "psyched up," as my grandchildren would say.

In order to "de-psyche" yourself regarding the temporary weight loss assistance for "crash" diets, examine the chart below. If you are still tempted to try the latest lose-ugly-fat-fast diet touted by the media as the means to painless overnight success, remember that the goal of dieting is fat loss, not dehydration. Since bodily fluids weigh about as much as body fat, scale changes reflect loss of fluids only, which is the phenomenon on which these low-carbohydrate diets are based.

Popular Weight Loss Fad Diets

Diet Plan	Brief Description	Our Comments
Advantage Diet System	Prepackaged meals (e.g., candy bars, canned pudding, canned stew) totalling 1,000 calories per day; 1-week supply costs $39.95	Monotonous, unappetizing and poorly balanced; does not help dieter to learn wise food selections.
Air Force Diet	Low-carbohydrate diet	Unbalanced, causes ketosis and other undesirable side effects; weight loss primarily due to water loss.
Anti-Cellulite Diets	Various low-calorie diets, plus potions and supplements	No such entity; cellulite is excess fat which can be lost on a sensible diet program.
Beverly Hills Diet	Fruit for 10 days, gradually adding other foods, but with certain types of food combinations avoided	Unbalanced, based on myths; serious side effects including diarrhea, dehydration, nutrient deficiencies.
Bio-Diet	Alternates "crash" diet with binges, plus supplements	Unhealthy practice; supplements do not provide weight loss benefits as claimed.
Cambridge Diet Plan	Very low-calorie liquid diet formula (330 calories per day)	Dangerously low in calories; serious side effects can damage health.
Dr. Atkin's Diet	Low-carbohydrate, high-protein diet	Unbalanced, high in fat/cholesterol causes ketosis and other serious side effects; weight loss due primarily to water loss.
Dr. Stillman's Quick Weight Loss Plan	Low-carbohydrate diet	Unbalanced, causes ketosis and other undesirable side effects; weight loss primarily due to water loss.
Drinking Man's Diet	Low-carbohydrate diet	Unbalanced, causes ketosis and other undesirable side effects; weight loss primarily due to water loss.
Fasting	Juices, teas and/or water only	Dangerous, unbalanced, effective only temporarily.
Fat-Destroyer Foods Diet	Low-carbohydrate, high-protein diet	Unbalanced, high in fat/cholesterol, causes

Popular Weight Loss Fad Diets

Diet Plan	Brief Description	Our Comments
		ketosis and other serious side effects; weight loss primarily due to water loss.
F-Plan Diet	Low-calorie, high fiber diet	May be deficient in calcium and undesirably high in fiber.
Fructose Diet	Low-carbohydrate diet, with relatively large intake of fructose	Fructose does not provide weight loss benefits claimed.
HCG Diet	Very low calorie diet with hormone injections	Injections do not provide weight loss benefits claimed.
I Love New York Diet	Alternates "crash" diet with binges	Unhealthy practice; promises unrealistic results.
Last Chance Diet	Very low-calorie liquid protein diet	Protein of poor quality; side effects include nutrient deficiencies, abnormal heartbeat, death.
Lecithin, Kelp, Vitamin B$_6$, and Vinegar Diet	Low-carbohydrate diet, plus supplements	Supplements do not provide weight loss benefits claimed.
Liquid Protein Diets	Formula with low-calorie intake plan	Protein may be poor quality; unbalanced; temporary at best, nutrient deficiencies can develop.
Mayo Diet	Grapefruit eaten before meals to "burn" fat	Ineffective, based on myth, successful only if calories are reduced.
Mono-Food Diets	E.g., cottage cheese and bananas, eggs and grapefruit, fruit only, etc.	Unbalanced, dull; temporary at best, nutrient deficiencies can develop.
Pritikin Diet	High-carbohydrate, high-fiber, low-fat diet	Unnecessarily restrictive and may be deficient in calcium, iron and other nutrients.
Protein-Sparing Diets	Very low-calorie diets requiring close medical supervision	Expensive; unbalanced, dangerous; only for morbidly obese.
Scarsdale Diet	High-protein diet	Unbalanced, potential for developing ketosis and nutrient deficiencies.
Ski Team Diet	Low-carbohydrate	Unbalanced, causes ketosis and other undesirable side effects;

Popular Weight Loss Fad Diets

Diet Plan	Brief Description	Our Comments
		weight loss primarily due to water loss.
Southampton Diet	Low-calorie diet with "mood foods"	Promises unrealistic results, promotes nutrition nonsense.
Starch Blocker Diet	Supposedly supplements block caloric contributions of starch foods	Ineffective; supplements (now illegal) can cause digestive disturbances.
Taller's "Calories-Don't-Count" Diet	Low-carbohydrate diet, plus safflower oil supplements	Supplements do not provide weight loss benefits claimed.
University Diet	Liquid protein diet	Unbalanced; temporary at best, nutrient deficiencies can develop.
Any more? Unfortunately yes.	More of the same nonsense.	Most likely unbalanced, dull, boring, and dangerous to your health, if you can even stick with it long enough!

Adapted from Stare and Aronson's *Your Basic Guide to Nutrition* (George F. Stickley Co, 1983).

What about the new diet programs which provide all the food you need for the day, but total less than 1000 calories (e.g., Genesis)?

These diet programs may offer well-balanced meals, but a daily caloric intake of less than 1000 calories will not provide you with the nutrients you need for good health. No matter what the advertisements for these programs claim, if your total caloric intake is too low, your body is unable to properly assimilate and utilize the nutrients you need for well-being.

Perhaps of greater importance, the prepared diet meal plans do nothing to teach dieters how to alter improper eating habits. By defining your total daily food intake, such diets eliminate your need to choose and thereby fail to assist you in developing menu planning skills. Once you halt the program and face the real world of food choices, you're on your own!

The only permanent way to lose weight is by changing undesirable eating behaviors—for good. Adoption of limited food plans, crash diets or other fads can only result in temporary weight loss, at best. So, be a wise consumer and a successful dieter: avoid fad diets in favor of an individualized, permanent, sensible weight control program based on the "Four-Prong Approach."

What do you think of the protein-sparing modified fast? I am a 55-year old male with over 100 pounds to lose.

Although the very restrictive medically supervised diets for the extremely overweight (with more than 100 pounds to lose) were once believed inappropriate for those over 50, this philosophy has been altered of late. Therefore, if your physician gives you the go-ahead, you may want to enroll in a medically supervised protein sparing modified fast program (PSMF). Although expensive, results are often encouraging for these diet programs.

The severely obese patients who adhere to PSMF diets are only allowed 6–8 ounces of high quality protein food per day, plus non-caloric liquids and nutritional supplements. Some lean body tissue is lost, but body fat stores can be substantially reduced. Since patients are under medical supervision, potential health dangers can be identified and curtailed. Such programs also offer behavior modification guidelines and careful introduction to normal eating patterns in the form of an individualized diet plan.

However, unsupervised PSMF diets—Total Image, the Cambridge Diet Plan, the fatal Last Chance Diet, and other home-use diets-in-a-cannister—can prove dangerous, and should never be adopted without close medical supervision. At an advancing age and with a significant amount of weight to lose, the only sensible plan is to obtain reliable, professional medical assistance.

Should I at least take a multivitamin/mineral supplement while I'm following the weight-loss plan?

Despite the deluge of advertisements which inform us that we need to take "nutritional insurance"—in the form of vitamin/mineral supplements—when dieting, exercising, under stress, or simply living in today's crazy world, there is no need to do so if your diet is well-balanced. Since you are including an adequate amount of a wide variety of foods from each of the Basic Four Food Groups, you are obtaining all of the nutrients your body needs.

Therefore, unless your physician prescribes a nutrition supplement due to a diagnosed deficiency, you need not waste your money in pharmacies and "health food" stores on unnecessary pills and potions. Spend the money at the supermarket for a delicious diet instead.

Once you lose those few extra pounds, you can gradually add more calories to your dietary intake by increasing portion sizes. Keep the weight off, however, by adjusting portion size to suit your needs and following an exercise plan. With a hearty appetite for activity, your body will reflect your youthful vigor instead of bearing that "rocking chair" spread.

Regular Physical Exercise

If I can't take in less calories and stay healthy, is there a healthful way to burn off more calories?

The best way to burn off those extra calories is by increasing your daily exercise level. Not only can you burn up calories as you are exerting yourself—bicycling, jogging even walking or swimming—but the added physical activity you undergo on a regular basis will also help to increase your overall metabolism so that you use more calories even when you aren't exercising. Thus, you'll be a fireball of energy all the time—and utilize calories galore! Add in the benefit of decreased appetite, and the benefit of physical activity for calorie counters is obvious. As part of the 4-prong program, regular physical exercise is an essential component in any longterm weight control program.

Although I'm in reasonably good health, I have not exercised for years. How can I start, and is it dangerous at my age?

Exercise—if too vigorous at the start, particularly in one not accustomed to physical activity—*can* be dangerous. Make sure to have a good physical examination by a physician before you begin any exercise program. If you receive a medically approved go-ahead, start gradually in working up to a full exercise program. Brisk walking is a good type of exercise for most who are getting along in years. You can start with a brief after-dinner walk in the evening, and progress to full-fledged daily hikes as you see fit. Regularity and intensity are essential, so don't just be a weekend stroller.

Do I need special equipment or clothing to embark on an exercise program?

The best foot forward can be made only if clad in a supportive shoe: Get yourself a sturdy pair of sneakers, running shoes, or hiking boots which have good soles and suit your exercise needs. This aspect of your fitness wardrobe is physically important, but psychologically it is helpful as well if you dress sharply: Brightly colored sneakers, sweatsuits, headbands/sweatbands, and other walking/jogging paraphernalia are available at reasonable prices. Attractive tennis outfits, swim suits, golf sweaters, and hats or caps are also widespread in sports shops and clothing stores. Warm winter wear is important, but bundling up need not be dowdy, for colorful hats, scarves, gloves, and warm-up suits add a glow to your sporting life. After all, if you look as if you enjoy the exercise, you may just find yourself loving it!

How can I keep myself from making excuses and avoiding exercise?

The best idea for one new to an exercise plan is to find a friend to "share the pain," as it seems to be at first. With an exercise "buddy" with whom to chat on walks, bicycle ride, go for a jog, or play tennis, golf, and other sports, the physical enjoyment may be enhanced, tedium reduced, and the chances of making excuses to avoid exercise are reduced. To get started on a responsible physical activity program, find youself a responsible partner. If he or she lacks motivation one day, you can be the "coach"—and vice versa. And once you have been following your exercise program for a while, you will probably find that you look forward to the physical activity. Many exercise enthusiasts are "addicted" to their daily bouts of energy expenditure. With time and persistence, you may discover that your program of physical activity is an integral and enjoyable component of your lifestyle—a healthful one, at that. More on exercises in the next chapter.

Tips on Behavioral Changes

What other lifestyle changes can help with weight loss?

Any change in lifestyle that requires you to move your body around more can help, for example: get in the habit of walking up 2 or 3 flights of stairs, rather than riding the escalator or waiting for the elevator; instead of driving around in search of the parking space closest to your destination, park several blocks away and walk; get off the bus a few blocks from your goal, and stride there briskly; and if you golf, instead of opting for the motorized cart, try to walk the course. In other words, on a daily basis you can increase your level of physical exercise in simple ways. Added to a regular program of daily exercise, the increased level of caloric output will help you to shed some pounds. And such a lifestyle change—from inactive to active—can boost your self-image and morale as well.

Another important lifestyle habit to alter in the attempt to maintain a reasonable weight is your individual eating pattern: if your food habits have led to undesired weight gain, then these need to be improved. Take the following quiz to examine your own eating habits and determine the changes you can make to ward off undesired eating/weight gain events:

Often	Occasionally	Never	
☐	☐	☐	1) Do you reward yourself with food?
☐	☐	☐	2) Do you feel guilty if you do not eat all of the food which you have been served?

☐ ☐ ☐ 3) Do you associate people, places, and events from the past with specific foods?

☐ ☐ ☐ 4) Does the sight of food make you feel hungry?

☐ ☐ ☐ 5) Does the smell of food make you feel hungry?

☐ ☐ ☐ 6) Does the thought of eating make you feel hungry?

☐ ☐ ☐ 7) Do you eat according to the clock (e.g., noontime automatically signifies lunch-time)?

☐ ☐ ☐ 8) Do you eat while simultaneously engaged in other activities (e.g., reading, watching television, working—job, house, school—talking on the phone, driving, etc.)?

☐ ☐ ☐ 9) Do you eat when you are emotionally stimulated (you turn to food when you are bored, frustrated, nervous, lonely, fatigued, depressed, happy, etc.)?

☐ ☐ ☐ 10) Do you put off or avoid unpleasant activities by eating instead?

☐ ☐ ☐ 11) Do you eat because of the influence of others (employer, family, spouse, parents, friends, etc.)?

☐ ☐ ☐ 12) Do you find yourself searching unsuccessfully for foods to satisfy unknown cravings?

In order to alter those habits which may have led to the upcreep of unwanted pounds, use the following questionnaire to begin lifestyle improvement:

1. Choose desirable alternatives to food for use as a reward. List some

   examples: _____

   _____

   _____

2. Leave one bite on your plate at each meal or snack—resist the temptation to "clean the plate." Are you successful at this exercise? ☐ Yes ☐ No

   ☐ Sometimes   Why or why not? _____

   _____

3. Whenever you are eating, ask yourself if it is by your own choice or trig-

gered by someone, someplace, or some event from your past. Briefly describe some of your conclusions: _____

_____

_____

4. Try not to eat in response to the sight of food; if you do so, briefly describe the event(s) and your feelings at the time: _____

_____

5. Try not to eat in response to the smell of food; if you do so, briefly describe the event(s) and your feelings at the time: _____

_____

_____

6. Avoid fantasizing about food; if you do find yourself fantasizing, briefly explain what you feel may have triggered your thoughts: _____

_____

7. Avoid eating according to the clock; if you are unsuccessful, list some examples of and possible reasons behind your failure(s): _____

_____

8. Avoid eating while engaged in other activities by making eating a sole experience. You can note your success, starting here: _____

_____

_____

9. Select alternative outlets for emotions. List some examples: _____

_____

_____

10. Avoid eating for the purpose of procrastination. When you must face an unpleasant task, do you usually: put it off? tackle the problem? eat instead? List some examples: _____

_____

11. Develop places other than the kitchen where you can seek refuge from people who stir up your food-related emotions to an undesirable degree.

List some of the places you may choose to utilize: _____

_____

12. Avoid dissatisfying searches for unknown foods. Whenever you are looking for a specific food to satisfy a particular craving, stop and reflect.

List your needs at the time: _____

_____

Are any of these needs edible? If not, do you really need to eat?
☐ Yes ☐ No

Describe your feelings on this: _____

_____

Remember: It took many years for you to establish your present eating habits, so don't expect to change these patterns overnight. With attention to your own needs and goals, plus patience with yourself as a human being, you can gradually alter your eating habits to fit your new, successful lifestyle.

I'm one of those unfortunate fatties who finds solace in my dinner plate. How can I break a habit I've indulged in for over 50 years?

It's tough after 50 years (or 30, 20, 10 or even just a short time) of eating too much, frequently drinking too much of alcoholic beverages, and/or avoiding exercise, to break such habits in order to adopt healthier lifestyle patterns. Eating is an emotional experience, foods have personal impact for many, and the psychological implications of altering one's diet are complex. If you really want to explore some of your own individual food/emotion behaviors, examine the checklist below—and your own responses:

RAISON D'ÊTRE, REASONS TO EAT

	YES	NO	SOMETIMES
1) Food tastes good and I simply love to eat.	☐	☐	☐
2) I overeat because I love to cook and I have to taste as I prepare.	☐	☐	☐
3) Eating "for free" means overeating (e.g., all-you-can-eat restaurants, parties, free samples, buffets, as a dinner guest, etc.)	☐	☐	☐
4) Traveling causes overeating, since there are places (i.e., restaurants) where it may be a once-in-a-lifetime visit (i.e., meal).	☐	☐	☐

5) Whenever food is present, it seems like my last chance to eat it, so I grab and gobble while I still can. ☐ ☐ ☐

6) I eat even when I'm not hungry just to be sure that I won't be hungry later. ☐ ☐ ☐

7) Television and snacking go hand-in-mouth. ☐ ☐ ☐

8) Eating is comforting, non-threatening, reassuring, and food is my "friend". ☐ ☐ ☐

9) I eat when my emotions are stirred— anger, fear, worry, joy, anything. ☐ ☐ ☐

10) If I'm bored, I turn to food. ☐ ☐ ☐

11) If I'm tired, I eat for energy. ☐ ☐ ☐

12) The start and completion of my latest "diet" signal me to overeat—for "the last time." ☐ ☐ ☐

13) Holidays mean food—lots of it, and plenty of leftovers on which to over-indulge for extended periods. ☐ ☐ ☐

14) I eat like a bird with others, and like a pig when no one is watching. ☐ ☐ ☐

15) Others often force/encourage/tempt/guilt-trip me into overeating. ☐ ☐ ☐

16) If I feel guilty, I eat—then I feel guilty about eating, too. ☐ ☐ ☐

Other reasons why I eat include: _____

Is there any way to pinpoint the unconscious habits one may have which are leading to overeating?

The most revealing method of examining your eating habits in order to uncover patterns requiring change is by maintaining a food intake record. If you write down what you eat right after you eat, and record associated information (including time of day, duration and location of meal/snack, eating companion(s) if any, degree of hunger, and emotions before and after eating), you can discover some of the unknown "cues" which trigger you to overeat, as well as any inappropriate eating habits which you have heretofore ignored or overlooked.

The Food Intake Record given below is a sample outline for designing an eating diary of your own. Try keeping track of your food intake in a similar diary—use a totable note pad which fits into pocket or purse—for several days, a week, or longer. You may find that the act of recording your food intake causes you to eat less because you are more conscious of what you are putting in your mouth. You might also discover that the eating record is a practical way to balance your diet, since you have in print just what you have eaten and can menu plan accordingly.

After recording your food intake for several days, examine your Food Intake Record carefully:

- Are there certain times of day when you tend to overeat? What are the associated emotions at these times?
- Do you gulp your food down in only a few minutes? Do you eat standing up in the kitchen or on the run?
- Are you an alone-eater, or do you overeat with certain people? Again, what are the associated emotions?
- How hungry *are* you when you eat a meal or snack? Are you eating for reasons other than physical hunger?

Of course, we all eat inappropriately once in awhile, but if you can pinpoint the eating trends which are contributing to your weight problem, you'll have made the first step toward changing your lifestyle—for the better.

Once I decide to really lose some weight—and keep it off—how can I determine the best weight for me? Don't say the weight at which I got married, because that was more than 40 years (and 4 grandchildren) ago!

Although the common terms used to define appropriate body weight are "ideal" and "desirable," these are misleading because there is no ideal weight for height—everyone is different, after all—and the weight one might desire is often unrealistic. Therefore, a better term is "reasonable weight": aim for a body weight *range* at which you would feel comfortable and which you can maintain without starving yourself. This need not be the weight at which you got married, nor your weight at age 18, 21, 30, 50, or even the illusive weight you aspired to attain all your life. As long as your weight goal is reasonable, attainable, comfortable, practical, and healthful, you should be able to reach and maintain this range—for a lifetime.

It is also a good idea to avoid the temptation of becoming a scale addict: weigh yourself once a week, without clothes, before breakfast. There is no need to weigh yourself every day, since body weight fluctuates greatly during the day due to shifts in bodily fluids. Why weigh yourself daily to determine weight loss results when the following influences can serve to mislead you by affecting the scale

FOOD INTAKE RECORD

Date & Time	Duration of Meal (minutes)	Food and Amount	Where Eaten*	With Whom**	Degree of Hunger***	Associated Emotions/ Comments****

*Standing, sitting, walking, kitchen, restaurant, friend's house, etc.
**Alone, spouse, child, friend, etc.
***0–not hungry or full 1–almost hungry 2–body is sending hunger messages 3–very hungry
****Boredom, tension, stress, loneliness, depression, etc.

weight you record: Food and drink in digestive tract; Salt (sodium) intake which can retain fluids; Humidity and exercise which affect fluid retention; Reliability of scales.

Some of the more reliable methods for determining body fat—since scale weight does not differentiate between body fat, fluids, and lean muscle tissue, so you may not be over*weight* but can still be over*fat*—include the following:

- Skinfold measurement—calipers measure the thickness of skin in certain body areas reflective of the overall degree of body fat;
- Pinch test—home method to determine your general degree of overfat by pinching the back arm skin midway between elbow and shoulder—can you pinch an inch or more?
- Mirror test—as unpleasant as it is revealing, this body fat reflection method simply entails standing naked in front of a full-length mirror and objectively examining your body—are there areas you want to trim down and/or firm up?
- Mathematical formulas—for males, 106 pounds for the first five feet of height plus 6 pounds for each additional inch, and for females, 100 pounds for the first five feet plus 5 pounds for each additional inch.

All of these methods, like the bathroom or doctor's scales, are merely guides to help you determine a reasonable weight range. It's your body and your lifestyle that will ultimately result in the weight at which you feel and look your best. NOTE: Many older individuals do not gain *weight* but, due to overall decrease in physical activity, gain body *fat*. Thus, the best method to control body fat, as well as weight, is through a regular program of physical activity.

How can I keep myself from making excuses and "pigging out," as my grandchildren call it?

The key to success in avoiding the strong temptations to dump your diet in favor of "pigging out" lies in allowing yourself to enjoy your favorite foods—in moderation. If you restrict yourself too severely, the tendency is to overreact, to rebel by overeating. However, if you avoid the "diet deprivation" syndrome and allow yourself to indulge (moderately), such undesirable behaviors can be avoided. After all, if you accept the fact that a homemade brownie for a snack or a glass of wine before dinner is allowable, you are less apt to go overboard. If you have convinced yourself that any temporary diversion from your diet plan is an all-or-nothing event, one which triggers high-calorie "pig-outs" followed by guilt, then you have not permanently altered your eating habits to suit a healthful lifestyle.

So if you want to really enjoy food as part of your long and healthy life, you need to allow yourself the freedom to do just that. And if you overdo (i.e., "pig out") on occasion, there is no need to condemn yourself for being human. Just examine why you indulged and accept your behavior. Why not go for a brisk walk afterward and burn off some of those indulgent calories? And bring the grandchildren along for added energy!

A New Lifestyle—Sizing Yourself Up

Are there other changes I need to make—even at this stage in the game—to enhance my new lifestyle?

There may be some additional lifestyle changes you will want to make in order to help to ensure a long and healthy life span. First take the brief quiz below by selecting the answers which typically suit your lifestyle:

YES	NO	
☐	☐	1) I get seven to eight hours of sleep every night.
☐	☐	2) I do not smoke cigarettes.
☐	☐	3) I drink alcohol in moderate amounts.
☐	☐	4) I exercise every day.
☐	☐	5) I eat breakfast every morning.
☐	☐	6) I eat regular meals every day.
☐	☐	7) I am at a reasonable weight.

If you were able to honestly answer *Yes* to all of the above statements, you probably have quite a healthy lifestyle. Congratulations!

However, if like most Americans, you had to answer *No* to more than one of the above statements, you may be cutting down your total life span! According to the results of a well-known study (conducted at UCLA in 1977 by Bellac and Breslow), men who adhere to six out of these seven "health habits" most of the time can expect to live 11 years longer (women can expect to live 7 years longer) than those who adhere to fewer than four!

Perhaps even more important than leading a healthy lifestyle, however, is enjoying life. If you are perfectly fit physically but emotionally barren, chances are good that you will not outlive George Burns. Yet, if you have a healthy *joie de vivre*, you may increase your life span—mostly because you are enjoying your life too much for it to end! Make your diet, exercise program, lifestyle habits and patterns, and outlook on life, fun and exciting—and you will probably be around a lot longer to enjoy it all.

How can I evaluate myself to determine whether my overall lifestyle is—finally!—a healthful one?

We like to suggest that individuals of all ages self-administer the U.S. Department of Health and Human Services HEALTH STYLE* quiz, with a few additional miscellaneous questions we consider pertinent as well. Take the self-test given below, eliminating any questions which are not relevant to your current individual lifestyle (e.g., if you do not drive, omit the first three SAFETY statements). Remember that this is not a pass-fail test, but can be used as a means of enlightening you as to your own lifestyle patterns which may need special attention. Health is not just the absence of disease, but a sense of well-being. Your health status is less a function of age as it is a reflection of how healthy your *lifestyle* is. It's never too late to be actively healthy!

	Almost Always	Sometimes	Almost Never
Cigarette Smoking			
If you never smoke, enter a score of 10 for this section and go to the next section on *Alcohol and Drugs.*			
1. I avoid smoking cigarettes.	2	1	0
2. I smoke only low tar and nicotine cigarettes *or* I smoke a pipe or cigars.	2	1	0
Smoking Score:			
Alcohol and Drugs			
1. I avoid drinking alcoholic beverages *or* I drink no more than 1 or 2 drinks a day.	4	1	0
2. I avoid using alcohol or other drugs (especially illegal drugs) as a way of handling stressful situations or the problems in my life.	2	1	0
3. I am careful not to drink alcohol when taking certain medicines (for example, medicine for sleeping, pain, colds, and allergies).	2	1	0
4. I read and follow the label directions when using prescribed and over-the-counter drugs.	2	1	0
Alcohol and Drugs Score:			

---

*DHHS Publication NO. (PHS) 81-50155, U.S. Government Printing Office, Washington, D.C., 1981.

Eating Habits

1. I eat a variety of foods each day, such as fruits and vegetables, whole grain breads and cereals, lean meats, low-fat dairy products, dry peas and beans.   4   1   0
2. I limit the amount of fat, saturated fat, and cholesterol I eat (including fat on meats, eggs, butter, cream, shortenings, and organ meats such as liver).   2   1   0
3. I limit the amount of salt I eat by cooking with only small amounts, not adding salt at the table, and avoiding salty snacks.   2   1   0
4. I avoid eating too much sugar (especially frequent snacks of sticky candy or soft drinks).   2   1   0

Eating Habits Score: _____

Exercise/Fitness

1. I maintain a reasonable weight, avoiding overweight and underweight.   3   1   0
2. I do vigorous exercises for 15–30 minutes at least 3 times a week (examples include jogging, swimming, brisk walking).   3   1   0
3. I do exercises that enhance my muscle tone for 15–30 minutes at least 3 times a week (examples include yoga and calisthenics).   2   1   0
4. I use part of my leisure time participating in individual, family, or team activities that increase my level of fitness (such as gardening, bowling, golf, and tennis).   2   1   0

Exercise/Fitness Score: _____

Stress Control

1. I have a job or do other work that I enjoy.   2   1   0
2. I find it easy to relax and express my feelings freely.   2   1   0
3. I recognize early, and prepare for, events or situations likely to be stressful for me.   2   1   0
4. I have close friends, relatives, or others whom I can talk to about personal matters and call on for help when needed.   2   1   0
5. I participate in group activities (such as church and community organizations) or hobbies that I enjoy.   2   1   0

Stress Control Score: _____

Safety

1. I wear a seat belt while riding in a car.	2	1	0
2. I avoid driving while under the influence of alcohol and other drugs.	2	1	0
3. I obey traffic rules and the speed limit when driving.	2	1	0
4. I am careful when using potentially harmful products or substances (such as household cleaners, poisons, and electrical devices).	2	1	0
5. I avoid smoking in bed.	2	1	0

Safety Score: _____

Miscellaneous

1. If I watch television, it is for an hour or less a day.	2	1	0
2. I interact with friends and/or family on a daily basis.	2	1	0
3. I learn new things every day, and try to keep up-to-date on local and world events.	2	1	0
4. I am careful with my prescription medications, and do not find that they cause me any mental confusion or dullness.	2	1	0
5. My attitude is youthful and vibrant, a reflection of my love of life.	2	1	0

Miscellaneous Score: _____

Your Healthstyle Scores

Cigarette Smoking	Alcohol & Drugs	Eating Habits	Exercise & Fitness	Stress Control	Safety	Miscellaneous
10	10	10	10	10	10	10
9	9	9	9	9	9	9
8	8	8	8	8	8	8
7	7	7	7	7	7	7
6	6	6	6	6	6	6
5	5	5	5	5	5	5
4	4	4	4	4	4	4
3	3	3	3	3	3	3
2	2	2	2	2	2	2
1	1	1	1	1	1	1
0	0	0	0	0	0	0

After you have figured your scores for each of the 7 sections, circle the number in each column that matches your score for that section of the test.

Remember, there is no total score for this test. Consider each section separately. You are trying to identify aspects of your lifestyle that you can improve in order to be healthier and to reduce the risk of illness. Let's see what your scores reveal.

WHAT YOUR SCORES MEAN TO YOU

Scores of 9 and 10

Excellent! Your answers show that you are aware of the importance of this area to your health. More important, you are putting your knowledge to work for you by practicing good health habits. As long as you continue to do so, this area should not pose a serious health risk. It's likely that you are setting an example for your family and friends to follow. Since you got a very high score on this part of the test, you may want to consider other areas where your scores indicate room for improvement.

Scores of 6 to 8

Your health practices in this area are good, but there is room for improvement. Look again at the items you answered with a "Sometimes" or "Almost Never." What changes can you make to improve your score? Even a small change can often help you achieve better health.

Scores of 3 to 5

Your health risks are showing! Would you like more information about the risks you are facing and about why it is important for you to change these behaviors? Perhaps you need help in deciding how to successfully make the changes you desire. In either case, help *is* available.

Scores of 0 to 2

Obviously, you were concerned enough about your health to take the test, but your answers show that you may be taking serious and unnecessary risks with your health. Perhaps you are not aware of the risks and what to do about them. You can easily get the information and help you need to improve, if you wish. The next step is up to you.

You Can Start Right Now!

In the test you just completed were numerous suggestions to help you reduce your risk of disease and premature death. Here are some of the most significant:

Avoid cigarettes

Cigarette smoking is the single most important preventable cause of illness and early death. It is especially risky for pregnant women and their unborn babies. Persons who stop smoking reduce their risk of getting heart disease and cancer. So if you're a cigarette smoker, think twice about lighting that next cigarette. If you choose to continue smoking, try decreasing the number of cigarettes you smoke and switching to a low tar and nicotine brand.

Follow sensible drinking habits

Alcohol produces changes in mood and behavior. Most people who drink are able to control their intake of alcohol and to avoid undesired, and often harmful, effects. Heavy, regular use of alcohol can lead to cirrhosis of the liver, a leading cause of death. Also, statistics clearly show that mixing drinking and driving is often the cause of fatal or crippling accidents. So if you drink, do it wisely and in moderation.

Use care in taking drugs

Today's greater use of drugs—both legal and illegal—is one of our most serious health risks. Even some drugs prescribed by your doctor can be dangerous if taken when drinking alcohol or before driving. Excessive or continued use of tranquilizers (or "pep pills") can cause physical and mental problems. Using or experimenting with illicit drugs such as marijuana, heroin, cocaine, and PCP may lead to a number of damaging effects or even death.

Eat sensibly

Overweight individuals are at greater risk for diabetes, gallbladder disease, and high blood pressure. So it makes good sense to maintain proper weight. But good eating habits also mean holding down the amount of fat (especially saturated fat), cholesterol, sugar and salt in your diet. If you must snack, try nibbling on fresh fruits and vegetables. You'll feel better—and look better, too.

Exercise regularly

Almost everyone can benefit from exercise—and there's some form of exercise almost everyone can do. (If you have any doubt, check first with your doctor.) Usually, as little as 15–30 minutes of vigorous exercise three times a week will help you have a healthier heart, eliminate excess weight, tone up sagging muscles, and sleep better! Think how much difference all these improvements could make in the way you feel!

Learn to handle stress

Stress is a normal part of living; everyone faces it to some degree. The causes of stress can be good or bad, desirable or undesirable (such as a promotion on the job or the loss of a spouse). Properly handled, stress need not be a problem. But unhealthy responses to stress—such as driving too fast or erratically, drinking too much, or prolonged anger or grief—can cause a variety of physical and mental problems. Even on a very busy day, find a few minutes to slow down and relax. Talking over a problem with someone you trust can often help you find a satisfactory solution. Learn to distinguish between things that are "worth fighting about" and things that are less important.

Be safety conscious

Think "safety first" at home, at work, at school, at play, and on the highway. Buckle seat belts and obey traffic rules. Keep poisons and weapons out of the reach of children, and keep emergency numbers by your telephone. When the unexpected happens, you'll be prepared.

Healthy Outlook—NOT Miscellaneous

It is essential to overall good health for you to limit your isolated time, and to use the alone-time well. This means avoiding TV-marathons, in favor of being socially active, keeping up with the world's happenings, and maintaining a keen mind. If your attitude towards life is healthy, and your lifestyle is equally healthful, your healthstyle will rate tops.

Dr. George Sheehan: Staying Trim without Dieting

An inspirational writer and lecturer, Dr. George Sheehan is a cardiologist and runner who has successfully combined his vocation with an avocation. In his best-selling books and popular lectures, Dr. Sheehan advises his audiences to adopt sensible eating habits and to adhere to a program of regular physical exercise. And he emphasizes the importance of enjoying exercise, so that fitness is a personal philosophy which is incorporated from within. As Dr. Sheehan points out in his newest book, *How to Feel Great 24 Hours a Day* (Simon and Schuster, 1983), "Your body reveals you within and without."

So how does Dr. Sheehan stay slim and fit, despite a hectic career which often necessitates long hours and wide travel? Does Dr. Sheehan resort to quick-loss diet tricks to keep in shape, or is he just plain fortunate physically, i.e., naturally slender?

Weighing in the same lean range as during his college years, Dr. Sheehan maintains his trim physique with a lifestyle which emphasizes adequate activity and careful diet planning. During his post-college era, Dr. Sheehan stopped running and was a good 25 pounds heavier. Over twenty years ago, however, Dr. Sheehan resumed his college running habits and redeveloped the fit body he still maintains today.

Dr. Sheehan does not encourage waist watchers to attempt marathon training, nor will he advocate a Spartan diet regime. While currently averaging around 30 minutes of daily running, Dr. Sheehan is careful to eat well to properly fuel his body for exercise. Moderation—in both exercise and diet—is the key.

Anyone who enjoys daily exercise can choose to emulate Dr. Sheehan's safe, sensible weight control plan sampled below. Better yet, however, is to develop a personal weight control plan which suits your individual needs and desires. Thus, you can allow your body to reveal *you*—both inside and out!

DR. SHEEHAN'S DIET PLAN—SAMPLE MENU

Big Breakfast—Juice, egg, potatoes, cereal and fruit, toast, skim milk, coffee
Light Lunch—Low-fat yogurt, beverage
Balanced Dinner—Vegetable soup, broiled fish, stir-fried vegetables, side-order pasta
Bedtime "Snack"—2 beers or non-alcoholic beers

DR. SHEEHAN'S EXERCISE PLAN

Running—3 hours per week
Weekends—races (5–10 miles)
Rest—1 day per week

Part III

Daily Special: Focusing on Fitness

DAILY SPECIAL: FOCUSING ON FITNESS

As the saying goes, people don't wear out as they age, they rust out! But this process is not necessarily an inevitable one. By treating your body like a valuable car, that is by sheltering it from the ravages of the environment and making sure to keep it tuned up, you can protect it from wearing out *and* rusting out. And by running you car—and exercising your body—every day, the premature aging of disuse can be avoided. Don't let your body get run down. Consider yourself a priceless antique car, a "limited edition" well worth preserving!

Advancing age need not indicate inactivity and infirmity. In fact, the older you get, the more important it becomes for you to be physically active. You may have entered the "golden years" with a solid background of years spent in various physical activities. This may provide you with strong physical resources to utilize in continued activity. Even if you have let yourself go, however, and have been out of shape for a while, you can still improve your physical fitness.

The level of physical fitness you attain—at any age—is determined by the amount of movement you are able and willing to make. Physical fitness (and health) can be defined as the condition of physical well-being which enables an individual to look and feel good, to successfully carry out any and all daily tasks, and to have enough energy left over for social and recreational activities with reserves capable of contending with emergency demands. In order to be physically fit, one must start with a supportive body state, that is, a well-nourished, disease-free *physical* being with adjustments made for any infirmities (e.g., hearing aid, eyeglasses, and dentures as required). To maintain the healthy body and become *fit*, one needs to incorporate regular physical activity into the pattern of living. An exercise program will lead to improvements in the following bodily functions: efficiency of heart and lungs, muscular strength and endurance, balance, flexibility, and coordination and agility.

The later years can be full of energy and excitement if you are physically fit. Achievement of a healthy level of fitness is possible, if you choose to work at it. The "golden years" need not be marred by a rusty body.

PROS AND CONS OF EXERCISE AFTER 50

Should someone over the age of 50 even try to engage in an exercise program?

Unless your physician advises against it, regular exercise may be even more beneficial to your health status now than ever before. Older people need not accept the myth that age brings on infirmity and inactivity. How we live our lives can predict our physical status: if we keep vital and active, so will our physical (and mental) selves. Anyone, at nearly any age, can improve physical fitness.

What exactly does "physical fitness" mean?

Physical fitness is the condition of overall well-being: "organic fitness" entails the maintenance of a well-nourished body free of disease or infirmities with any necessary adjustments for irreversible physical conditions (e.g., dentures, eyeglasses, hearing aid, etc.); "dynamic fitness" includes the capability for energetic, vigorous movement, so it requires efficiency of the heart and lungs, muscular strength and endurance, balance, flexibility, coordination and agility. If you are physically fit, you look healthy, you feel good, you can conduct activities of daily living without difficulty, and still have energy left both to enjoy any social, cultural, and/or recreational interests you may have and to fulfill any unusual demands which may arise.

How do I even begin on an exercise program?

The first step is to obtain your physician's approval. If you have any underlying health conditions which preclude rigorous exercise, your doctor will advise you as to the best alternative. If your health is acceptable, merely in need of the improvement to which regular exercise can lead, then your physician will give you the go-ahead (probably with much enthusiasm) to begin on an exercise program.

One of the best and simplest forms of exercise—which is often overlooked—is walking. It is certainly the most practical type of physical activity, one which almost anyone can enjoy. It also requires little in the way of financial expenditure for special equipment: a good sturdy pair of hiking shoes or running (sneaker-type) shoes plus some thick athletic socks are really all that may be required; in inclement weather, appropriate dress is also necessary. Then you need only select one or more walking routes which are safe, accessible, and pleasant.

If you think you may enjoy other forms of exercise, you might want to investigate the opportunities available in your area. Sports clubs, fitness centers, YMCA/YWCA's often provide older citizens with benefits and may set aside special times or classes for individuals over 50. Swimming, tennis, racquetball and squash, and even bicycling or jogging may prove to be *your* sport. It is essential, however, that you select an activity which you truly enjoy, or chances are good that you will not adhere to your exercise program for very long.

Start slowly, very slowly if you have been sedentary for a considerable length of time. Don't overdo, or you may be turned off by exercise—or even worse, you might hurt yourself and thereby interfere with any further physical activity. Try not to strain yourself, but do work up a sweat. You want to "huff and puff," but not "blow your house down"!

Plan a regular routine which you know you can adhere to, and then do it. You may soon be unable to stop!

What are the positive benefits of regular exercise, other than weight control?

Research indicates that exercise helps you to look, feel, and work better. Various bodily organs work more efficiently when you are exercising regularly. The digestive tract in particular becomes more efficient due to improved muscle tone so there should be fewer constipation woes once you are physically fit! Your cardiovascular and respiratory systems can also function at an improved level, your posture may improve, the pain of arthritis might lessen or even disappear. As body weight reaches a reasonable level, the disorders associated with overweight will diminish and/or fail to appear. Stronger muscles mean more overall physical strength and energy with reduced susceptibility to infection and disease, and more rapid recovery from illnesses or accidents. Rehabilitation and chances for survival are improved with physical fitness.

Although exercise does not prevent stress (nothing seems to do this in the stressful world we live in), being physically fit can help you to cope better with stressful events. Physical activity helps to reduce mental fatigue, ease tension, relax the nerves, and alleviate the boredom and depression which may accompany a sedentary lifestyle. By becoming physically fit, you will find that your self-image is improved, your self-confidence increases, and your attractiveness is enhanced. All this creates the environment required for developing a positive outlook, the love of life leading to a happy, long, healthful life.

Are there any negative aspects of regular exercise—besides the fact that we older folks are naturally prone to being seated?

At any age, sports-related injuries can occur. This is why it is important to avoid overdoing it, to begin slowly and gradually develop your level of fitness, and to follow a sensible exercise program. If you do hurt yourself, it is a wise idea to see a physician promptly. You may want to find out in advance if there is a reputable sports medicine clinic in your area which can provide affordable and dependable medical assistance if you ever happen to require it. Hopefully, you won't need to seek such services.

Are some activities better to undertake than others?

Your best bet is to adopt an exercise program which includes so-called "aerobic" activities. Aerobic exercises are those which require more oxygen for prolonged periods and thereby help the body in becoming more efficient in handling oxygen. Aerobic activities are endurance exercises but do not have to involve speed: walking, jogging, swimming, ice or roller skating, cross-country skiing, and bicycling are all examples of aerobic exercise.

It is also a good idea to include activities in your exercise program which you personally enjoy: bowling, golf, tennis and other sports can enhance your social joys as well as your physical health. A balance of aerobic exercise (for 20 to 30 minutes, 3 to 4 times a week) with other sports of individual preference can produce a physical activity plan you can adhere to for a healthy lifetime.

DEVISING AN INDIVIDUALIZED ACTIVITY PLAN

How can I incorporate some physical activity into my present "rocking chair" lifestyle?

The first step is to obtain the "go-ahead" from your physician. Even if you consider yourself to be a strong and healthy (albeit sedentary) oldster, it is essential that your doctor be supportive of your activity plan. It may be a good time to get your annual check-up anyway.

Have your physician help you select the appropriate level for daily exercise from the RED-WHITE-BLUE,* a series of "reasonable" exercises combined to provide a balanced daily workout which allows easy progression for gradually improved fitness. Created by specialists in designing activity programs for the older adult, one of the RED-WHITE-BLUE daily exercise plans should suit your present level of fitness. Keep in mind the fact that it is important to increase your level of fitness gradually by avoiding the urge to do too much too quickly. This usually results in discomfort, disappointment, and distaste for exercise, if not outright injury.

Must I do the Daily Exercise every day, or can I substitute alternative activities, such as gardening?

Gardening is usually not a "huffing and puffing" exercise, but you can substitute other activities for the RED-WHITE-BLUE exercise program which are more equivalent to your Daily Exercise workout.

---

*For a copy of this Plan write to the Superintendent of Documents, U.S. Government Printing Office, Washington, DC 20402; ask for Fitness Challenge in the Later Years (DHEW #DHD 75-20802, $3.50 per copy).

Taking a long hike, swimming, or going for a bike ride are acceptable replacements. Recreational activities such as fishing, horseshoes, ping-pong, shuffleboard, or gardening are fine to practice if you enjoy them, but should be added to—instead of substituted for—exercise.

What can I do to keep myself motivated to follow my activity plan?

One good method to make sure that you adhere to your Daily Exercise program is the "buddy system": find a partner to exercise with, and you will be able to support each other. If you are not "in the mood," your partner may motivate you, and vice versa. You may even get a whole group together—this might even enhance your social life as well as your level of physical fitness!

How to Enjoy Exercise and Avoid Gimmicks

Are there any practical tips so that I can increase my daily activity level in general?

Good idea! In addition to a Daily Exercise program and recreational activities, you can keep your body active throughout the day by stepping up your overall level of activity. The following tips may assist you in doing so:

- Walk instead of ride—whenever feasible, stretch your legs instead of traveling seated; get off the bus a few blocks before your intended destination and walk, and park your car in the far corner of the lot instead of the doorway.
- Take the stairs for two to four flights—instead of using elevators and escalators, give your heart and limbs a workout by climbing to your destination, or at least part-way.
- Find busy work that keeps your body active: chop wood, build a birdhouse, paint a fence, revamp your kitchen, do the house-cleaning, plant a garden, rake the leaves, mow the lawn, clean out the attic, go for a nature walk, etc.

Look for every possible opportunity to move your body. In no time at all, your "rocking chair" mentality will have been replaced with the more youthful vim and vigor which accompanies physical fitness and overall well-being.

Are there any exercises which older people should avoid?

When it comes to physical activity, you are your own best judge: select only those exercises which you can handle without overexerting or straining yourself. (And, of course, avoid any activities your physician advises against.) Like your dietary likes and dislikes, you should include those activities you enjoy and avoid those of personal disinterest. However, sometimes when you try a new food or beverage, you find that you like it a lot more than you thought. This can prove true with exercise. So, be adventurous. You may find that you are a natural at jogging when you had originally believed that a brisk walk was the extent of your physical capabilities.

It is also wise to avoid the many exercise gimmicks and health/fitness rip-offs which are currently flooding the shelves of sporting goods stores and "health food" shops. Such devices are cleverly promoted and advertised extensively in tabloids and magazines, yet are a waste of your money and of limited benefit to your health.

What are some examples of exercise gadgets which are only gimmicks?

Although the list is extensive and grows longer daily, some examples of the more popular non-exercises include:

- *Passive exercise machines*—the belts that vibrate you, rollers that pound you, and bicycles which pedal for you and thus require little effort on your part are ineffective forms of "exercise."
- *Spot reducers*—the rubber stretchers, reducing creams, and simple calisthenic aids and guides can only reduce you effectively in one spot—your wallet; spot-reducing is an invalid premise. An exercise/diet program will reduce fat stores all over; limiting the muscles you exercise to one area will reduce both the calories burned and the number of muscles strengthened.
- *Saunas, body wraps, rubber suits, and heat belts*—you may sweat more, but you will neither lose more body fat nor improve your physical fitness by using these gadgets; the only effective sweating is that which accompanies vigorous "huffing and puffing" exercises.

There are so many other gimmicks that it would take too much space to list them all. Just keep in mind that, as with fad diets and food frauds, caveat emptor: if it costs money and sounds too good to be true, it probably isn't worth the expenditure.

Do I need to take special nutrient supplements, now that I exercise every day?

Another gimmick touted to the gullible consumer is the necessity for taking food supplements. As explained in Part 1, a well-balanced diet which includes a wide variety of foods chosen from the Basic Four Groups can include all of the nutrients essential for good health. Daily exercise will enhance your health without elevating your nutrient needs to levels requiring supplementation.

Protein powders are the most common form of food supplement promoted to athletes. Yet, exercise does not increase protein needs and muscle-building does not necessitate supplementary protein! Most Americans consume two to three times the protein their bodies require anyway, so protein needs are easily met whether you are sedentary, active, or an athlete.

Vitamin and mineral supplements are also advertised as important for the physically active individual. However, exercise does not significantly increase your need for most of the 50 or so essential nutrients, and the slight rise in the requirement for certain B-vitamins is easily met by a dietary intake rich in carbohydrates. Thus, if your diet is well-balanced, you need not waste money on unnecessary food supplements—whether you are active or inactive—and if your diet is not well-balanced, it would be preferable to improve it, rather than resorting to the undesirable pattern of pill-popping.

Remember, too, that too much of some supplements has the potential for damaging health: protein powders can tax the kidneys and lead to protein imbalance; megadoses of water-soluble vitamins can produce serious side-effects; while certain minerals and fat-soluble vitamin overdoses can prove fatal. Obviously, if you are improving your health by exercising every day, you don't want to defeat your endeavors by throwing your nutritional balance out of kilter.

Is there any need, then, to alter my diet, now that I'm a senior athlete?

Not radically—so long as it is well-balanced, and includes enough food to provide the calories you need for energy and to maintain a reasonable weight. If you find that you are losing too much weight, you may want to increase your caloric intake to balance your newly expanded energy output: add in more complex carbohydrates such as breads, cereals, pastas, fruits, and vegetables, which will provide the extra B-vitamins you may need now that your caloric needs have increased.

Fluid losses are important to replace. Unfortunately, thirst is not an accurate indicator of fluid needs. If your exercise program is of the "huffing and puffing" variety—as it should be—you will need to be sure to drink plenty of fluids, at least two or even more quarts on exercise days. The beverage of choice is cool water, but fluid needs can be met with inclusion of such drinks as fruit juices, vegetable juices, milk, milkshakes, yogurt drinks, soft drinks, diet soft drinks, coffee, tea, and even some beer (note that the last three items tend to dehydrate, so are not advisable choices just after exercise).

Sodium losses from sweating can easily be replaced via the diet. Salt tablets are not safe, because they can cause gastric distress, sodium imbalance and dehydration. Most Americans consume too much salt (sodium) anyway, so any heavy losses during exercise are easily replaced. If you think you may have depleted your bodily sodium supplies this way, use a few extra shakes of the salt shaker.

Iron losses do occur in athletes, of particular importance for endurance athletes. If you are a marathoner or triathlete, you should check with your physician to determine the need for supplementation. Otherwise, a well-balanced diet—occasionally using lean red meats and liver—should be sufficient for your iron needs, as well as your other nutrient requirements, energy supply, and overall health.

Will my Daily Exercise plan and new level of increased physical activity help me to have an even longer life span?

Although research is still inconclusive as to whether regular physical activity can increase the *quantity* of years you live, it will certainly enhance the *quality* of your life. By adopting a regular program of exercise and increasing your level of physical fitness, you will soon find that, along with your improved dietary patterns, your healthful lifestyle is rewarding, physically and emotionally.

NOTE: One of the many benefits of physical fitness is the reduction of stress. Emotional stress can reduce the body's ability to ward off disease. According to a Harvard colleague, Dr. Herbert Benson, well-known author of books about stress, personality also plays a role in the prevention of illness and response to stress. "Not only does stress affect one's ability to fight disease, but how one interprets the stressful situation, as determined by one's personality, is important. What stresses one person may not stress another because we're all different," says Dr. Benson.

How are you holding up under the deluge of today's daily stresses? Try a brief self-analysis by answering the questions in the following checklist as honestly as possible.

Often	Sometimes	Never	
☐	☐	☐	Do you feel emotionally drained?
☐	☐	☐	Are you nervous and "up-tight"?
☐	☐	☐	Are you irritated by trivial matters?
☐	☐	☐	Do you feel physically tired and dragged out?
☐	☐	☐	Do you have trouble falling asleep?
☐	☐	☐	Do you find it difficult to concentrate for any length of time?
☐	☐	☐	Do you find that your memory is poor?

☐	☐	☐	Do you find it difficult to make even a simple decision?
☐	☐	☐	Do you become depressed for indefinable reasons?
☐	☐	☐	Have you lost interest in short- and long-range endeavors?

Thus, if you tend to get "up-tight" easily and find that the daily stresses of modern living are detracting from your physical and emotional well-being, your daily exercise plan should prove to be of great help. You may find that you need to incorporate other methods of stress reduction into your lifestyle as well. If you found yourself answering *Often* or *Sometimes* to most of the questions in the checklist, you might want to invest in one of the stress reduction programs available to the public. The local newspaper and your area hospital's dietary/mental health departments may list stress reduction programs—which are given free or for a minimal fee—under such titles as:

- Transcendental Meditation (TM)
- Yoga
- Hypnosis
- Exercises-for-relaxation courses
- Stress-relaxation courses

If you are physically fit, stress will be another aspect of your life which you are able to cope with healthfully. A sound diet, a fit body, and a relaxed attitude can make your later years among the best years of your life.

Dr. Benjamin Spock: Staying Active

Dr. Spock has long served as a household name, representing a philosophy of which most of today's parents, grandparents, and now-grown children are well aware. Often controversial and always outspoken, Dr. Benjamin Spock is still nationally recognized and respected as a lively spokesperson for a variety of issues of the American Lifestyle—from infant care and child-rearing practices to teen-age rebellion and elderly rights—and he stays actively involved in the lively politics of public debate. At age 81, Dr. Spock does not hesitate to become an integral contributor to the ongoing and energizing activities of our changing American culture.

What fuels the rapid pace set by Dr. Spock? Does he rely on fancy foods or special nutrition products to keep him on-the-go, looking fit and trim, ready to face his hectic schedule filled with lecturing, writing and travel? In keeping with his practical advice to the general public, Dr. Spock adheres to a sensible lifestyle pattern himself—including a healthful diet and hearty exercise routine.

Dr. Spock's diet is low in fat and focuses on whole grain cereals, fresh fruits, thick vegetable soups, stir-fried vegetables, and an occasional serving of chicken or fish. In marrying his vegetarian wife, Dr. Spock was converted—at age 73—to his current semi-vegetarian lifestyle. But Dr. Spock is not a dietary "purist," and his diet is based on the variety available in local supermarkets. He also confesses that he enjoys drinking beer!

There is no need for strict diets or crash weight loss plans, despite Dr. Spock's penchant for high-calorie brews. An avid boatsman, Dr. Spock spends half of each year in Arkansas, where he can be found rowing his single scull. Wintertime finds him in tropical climates where he enjoys snorkeling and sailing. No wonder he finds cold beer to be so refreshing!

Dr. Spock is living proof that fitness after 50 can mean a lifestyle which allows for the active pursuit of career, homelife, and just plain enjoyment in living. A sensible diet and regular physical exercise can only contribute to the pleasures of living a long and healthy life.

Irving Stone

Author and biographer, Irving Stone attributes his healthy longevity to abstinence rather than diet: "Unlike the people who live to eat, I eat merely to generate the strength to get a good day's work done. My four years in college boarding houses and fraternities also offered mediocre food, and so I never really got attached to the eating process. Besides, I can eat very little in the morning because I have to go to work; and I can eat very little at lunch because I have to go back to work; and at night I'm too damned tired to eat anything much even though I don't have to go back to work. My eating—or non-eating habits—are the bane of my family's life. Perhaps my abstinence is why I've stayed so healthy and energetic through my 80th birthday."

Perhaps his good health is due more to his extremely well-balanced diet, which emphasizes a variety of low-fat foods, adherence to his physician's individualized dietary advice, and an admirable exercise regimen that alternates ½–1 hour of daily swimming in the good weather with "very fast" walking in the hills behind his Beverly Hills home during the colder months of the year. And a "lust for life," if not for food, has certainly enhanced Mr. Stone's healthful lifestyle.

Part IV

Side Dishes: Special Problems in the Later Years

Governor Averell Harriman

Because he disliked questionnaires, long-time Presidential advisor W. Averell Harriman had his assistant provide information on his dietary habits when he was a 75-yr.-old politician. A well-balanced eater, Mr. Harriman included considerable amounts of fresh fruits and vegetables in his daily diet, ate high-quality protein and fiber-rich grains at each meal and enjoyed a moderate amount of alcohol as a glass of Scotch before dinner and a glass of wine with the evening meal. He worked up his healthy appetite for food and drink by swimming for thirty minutes every day.

SIDE DISHES: SPECIAL PROBLEMS
IN THE LATER YEARS

Aging is the genetic process which causes gradual deterioration of the body's cells. As you grow older, cell metabolism weakens and cells lose their ability to function: the rate of nerve impulse transmission slows, protein tissue is replaced with fat, and the senses are dulled. Your environment can further the aging process via stress, such as that imposed by: excessively hot weather, excessively cold weather, physically demanding labor, disease conditions, malnutrition, prolonged immobility, and lack of stimulation.

Yet, even in a temperate, supportive environment, cellular changes occur which eventually lead to the deterioration we know as "aging," as the cells which are dependent on nonfunctioning cells cease to function, and the organs they comprise begin to falter. If science could discover a means for cells to replenish themselves, you might be able to extend your "golden years" indefinitely!

Unfortunately, you probably will not even live a significantly longer life span than did your Biblical forebears. During the past several decades, there has not been much of an increase in life expectancy for those individuals who reach the age of twenty. Pharmacological advancements and medical developments have resulted in a reduced mortality rate for infants, but the death rates for diseases in other age groups have risen simultaneously. Therefore, more individuals can now live into adulthood, but most men live just beyond the 70th birthday, and the majority of females only outlast their male peers by around seven years.

Fortunately, advancements in the *quality* of life have exceeded scientific progress toward an extension in the *quantity* of life. You can really enjoy your "golden years" in this country due to the expansion of available health services, significant improvements in living standards, and notable advances in the fields of medicine and nutrition. Because of the increasing numbers of older citizens, public interest in the physical and psychosocial implications of aging has also grown.

Do you think you are currently in poor health due to your age? Perhaps your lack of youthful vitality is caused more by an inadequate diet than by your advancing years. Examine the chart below to pinpoint nutrition-related physical signs which you may have begun to notice as you entered the "golden years"—or perhaps even earlier on, in your "salad days" (see Table 4-1: Physical Signs of Malnutrition).

Physical problems from which you may be suffering might prove to be more diet-related than age-related. Poor oral health, sensory changes, digestive disturbances, fatigue, even so-called "senility," can

Table 4-1: Physical Signs of Malnutrition*

Body Area	Normal Appearance	Signs Associated with Malnutrition
Hair	Shiny; firm; not easily plucked.	Lack of natural shine; hair dull and dry; thin and sparse; can be easily plucked.
Face	Skin color uniform; smooth, pink, healthy appearance; not swollen.	Skin color loss; skin dark over cheeks and under eyes; lumpiness or flakiness of skin of nose and mouth; swollen face; enlarged glands; scaling of skin around nostrils.
Eyes	Bright, clear, shiny; no sores at corners of eyelids; membranes a healthy pink and are moist; no prominent blood vessels or mound of tissue.	Eye membranes are pale; redness of membranes; redness of eyelid corners; dryness of eye membranes; cornea (transparent outer coat of eyeball) has dull appearance; cornea is soft; scar on cornea; ring of fine blood vessels around cornea.
Lips	Smooth, not chapped or swollen.	Redness and swelling of mouth or lips, especially at corners of mouth.
Tongue	Deep red in appearance; not swollen or smooth.	Swelling; scarlet and raw tongue; magenta (purplish color) of tongue; smooth tongue; swollen sores.
Teeth	No cavities; no pain; bright.	May be missing; gray or black spots; cavities (caries).
Gums	Healthy; red; do not bleed; not swollen.	"Spongy" and bleed easily; recession of gums.
Glands	Face not swollen.	Thyroid enlargement (front of neck); parotid enlargement (cheeks become swollen).
Skin	No signs of rashes, swellings, dark or light spots.	Dryness of skin; sandpaper feel of skin; flakiness of skin; skin swollen and dark; red swollen pigmentation of exposed areas; excessive lightness or darkness of skin; black and blue marks due to skin bleeding; lack of fat under skin.
Nails	Firm, pink.	Nails are spoon-shaped; brittle; ridged nails.
Muscular and skeletal systems	Good muscle tone; some fat under skin; can walk or run without pain.	Muscles have "wasted" appearance; person cannot get up or walk properly; bones easily broken.
Internal Systems		
Cardiovascular	Normal heart rate and rhythm; no murmurs or abnormal rhythms; normal blood pressure for age.	Rapid heart rate; abnormal rhythm; elevated blood pressure.
Gastro-intestinal	No palpable organs or masses.	Liver enlargement; enlargement of spleen (usually indicates other associated diseases); digestive disturbances.
Nervous	Psychological stability; normal reflexes.	Mental irritability and confusion; burning and tingling of hands and feet; loss of position and vibratory sense (balance); weakness and tenderness of muscles (may result in inability to walk); decrease and loss of ankle and knee reflexes.

*Adapted from "Nutritional Assessment in Health Programs, Part I." *American Journal of Public Health* (63), Nov., 1973, p. 18.

be influenced by diet patterns, and by lifestyles in general. Chronic diseases often entail dietary treatment, and the role of nutrition as a preventive factor is currently undergoing much research. There are some specific dietary do's and don'ts, however, that you may want to heed in order to help your later years really sparkle.

Are there dietary changes I can make so that I'll feel 30 (or more!) years younger?

You may be able to remember how you used to feel 30-plus years ago: You may have tired less readily, needed less sleep, had a better appetite, been more active physically, and perhaps even worried less about life's stresses and strains. Yet vitality is not the sole possession of youth, nor need it be discovered in a fountain or purchased in an elixir bottle. You can feel thirty years younger—or more—if you maintain a youthful outlook. A healthy body can assist you in attaining a vital emotional energy level as well.

Diet, of course, is one aspect of your lifestyle which you can alter in order to improve your state of health. Although you may hear claims to the contrary, there is no need to grab for food supplements in an attempt to invigorate: Like the anti-aging cremes and schemes, nutritional manipulations for prolonging youth are bottled sales gimmicks, used merely to generate income for pseudoscientists. As an aware consumer, however, you need not fall for fountain-of-youth diet claims. Instead, you can utilize your nutrition knowhow to adopt a dietary pattern which is conducive to good health, provides the nutrients and energy you need, and helps you feel young and alive.

A well-balanced diet which includes a wide variety of foods from each of the Basic Four Food Groups is the best pattern to follow—at any age. If you have some excess poundage to shed, doing so will certainly add life to your years—as well as add years to your life. By keeping portion sizes moderate and watching out for fat-calories, a diet emphasizing fruits, vegetables, grains, legumes, low-fat milk products and lean meats can provide you with the nutrients and energy you need to maintain a healthy body at a reasonable weight.

Alcoholic beverages used in moderation may also add to your life span, and to your enjoyment of it. Excessive drinking, however, can only cut your life short. And cigarette smoking will put a serious damper on your lifestyle, ruining health, speeding up aging, and robbing you of years of life. Unlike eating and drinking, cigarette smoking should not be indulged in even on a moderate scale. If you smoke cigarettes, stop. Even if you are one of those individuals who has smoked for decades without fear, you should face the facts: *You are playing with fire.*

To feel young, be young: eat healthfully, drink moderately, be active physically and socially, and don't ever put another cigarette into your mouth. You'll have a lot more years of smiling to enjoy.

COMMON ILLS AFFECTED BY NUTRITION

Speaking of smiling, isn't it a normal process of aging to need dentures?

Happily, no. Although a significant percentage of adults do lose some or all of their teeth (by age 60, half of all Americans have lost their teeth, two-thirds by age 75), this is not an inevitable circumstance, but a preventable occurrence. With good dental hygiene—conscientious brushing after meals and daily flossing of teeth—and regular check-ups with your dentist, oral health can be maintained throughout your life. Diet, too, plays a role in dental care, because tooth decay can be kept to a minimum if in-between meal snacks do not include sticky sweets (chewy candies, toffees, gum, dried fruits, etc).

Recent research indicates that any carbohydrate (sugar or starch) which is allowed to remain on tooth surfaces can contribute to the development of tooth decay. So dietary composition may really prove less important than the tooth brushing which follows food consumption.

Healthy gums free of disease can help to support teeth throughout life. A well-balanced diet which includes plenty of fruits and vegetables will assist in the maintenance of healthy gums. Gum disease (gingivitis and periodontitis) is usually the result of years of poor dental hygiene and a poor diet. So the loss of teeth which necessitates dentures is less a process of aging than an event which occurs later in life once the ill practices of years behind finally catch up.

If you do have dentures for these or other reasons, there is no need to restrict food intake to bland, puréed dietary fare. When dentures are fitted properly, you should be able to enjoy just about everything the non-denture wearer can eat. On occasions when gums become inflamed or sore, simply eat soft non-spicy foods for a while until the irritation dies down. Just as dentures do not inevitably accompany the aging process, neither does wearing dentures require a lifelong blenderized diet. Fortunately, the need for dentures should become less common in the years to come due to the fluoridation of public water supplies which was greatly increased 25 to 30 years ago: Fluoridation not only decreases tooth decay by 60 to 70%, but this essential process helps to lessen the incidence of periodontal disease, loss of teeth in adult life, and ultimately the need for dentures.

Is there any kind of nutrition supplement available to treat gum disease?

Gum disease (gingivitis and periodontal disease) is best *prevented* by good dental hygiene, a well-balanced diet, fluoridation and regular visits to a dentist. Taking nutritional supplements after you have developed gum disease is a waste of your money, time, and hopes. A good periodontist can effectively treat the gum disease, and should not prescribe supplements of vitamins or minerals unless you have a diagnosed deficiency. NOTE: Older Americans tend to have intakes of vitamin C which are low to inadequate. Although taking large doses of vitamin C is unwise, healthy gums do require adequate dietary inclusion of foodstuffs rich in this vitamin. Therefore, be sure to include a daily serving of citrus fruit, tomato juice, fresh melon or strawberries, cabbage or broccoli or other sources of vitamin C—for the health of your oral cavity, as well as for the rest of your body, and to acquire the additional nutritional benefits such foods provide.

Is it a normal process of aging to lose one's sense of taste? Ever since I turned grey, I have had to douse all my meals with seasonings, or everything tastes blah!

All of our senses, including those of taste and smell, tend to become dulled with age. It is unknown whether this process is part of the biological changes which occur with aging, or whether environmental influences such as diet may have an effect. For example, older individuals tend to have marginal intakes of the mineral zinc, a deficiency of which causes decreased taste acuity. However, this does not mean that you should take zinc supplements—or any other nutritional aids—unless physician-prescribed. Until there is more evidence to indicate dietary manipulations which can sharpen our senses, your best bet is to adhere to a well-balanced, well-seasoned diet.

Sometimes, it is less that your senses are dulled, but more that your diet is drab: Do you overcook vegetables until mushy? Rely only on the same canned fruits, white bread, corn flakes and hamburger every day? Or is your diet filled with new food flavors, varying textures, spices and herbs, freshly cooked and freshly baked foodstuffs? There certainly is nothing wrong with seasoning your foods—unless you are salting them heavily, which is an undesirable practice, especially if you are prone to high blood pressure—but you may find that if you spice up your diet with new, flavorful foods, your senses will reawaken. NOTE: Turning grey has nothing to do with losing taste and smell acuity, but is a matter of heredity.

How can I get my 81-year-old mother to eat? She's losing weight, but never can work up much of an appetite.

That is frequently a difficult problem, all too common in the elderly. Smaller portions, attractive colorful foods, a pleasant, and cheerful atmosphere free from "nagging" about eating can do wonders to stimulate food consumption. Also, a glass of wine before meals may help to awaken the appetite.

If your mother is capable, physical activity can help her to feel more like eating. So will outside interests and mental stimulation. Sitting around in a chair all day, gazing and dozing, often leads to lack of appetite for food and anything else life has to offer. With zest for living, your mother may rediscover eating enjoyment as well.

My father-in-law stopped eating cheese over ten years ago because he claims that it "binds him up," but he still takes laxatives almost daily. Is there something else he should be eliminating from his diet?

First of all, the old myth that cheese is "binding" is simply that—an old myth. Most cheeses are moderately high in fat, so are digested more slowly than foods low in fat. Cheese doesn't contain any fiber, which helps to speed the digestive process. But cheese is certainly not guilty as charged, and is a good source of calcium to contribute strength to your father-in-law's aging bones.

Laxative abuse, on the other hand, should be discouraged. In the quest for "regularity," many people resort to the use of various medicinals which stimulate or aid elimination. However, chronic use of these drugs can result in a host of undesirable side effects, including the inability to be "regular" without them. Therefore, it is the intake of laxatives which should be eliminated!

Why not use "nature's laxatives" instead? Foods which contain fiber can be considered "nature's laxatives," since fiber is largely indigestible and helps to stimulate digestion. This process is beneficial to the overall health of the digestive system, so that adequate fiber in the diet will:

- increase bulk so that larger, softer stools are produced on a more frequent basis;
- decrease the amount of time undigested foods spend in the intestines; and
- decrease straining with elimination.

The possible health benefits associated with these changes include:

- alleviation and prevention of constipation;
- decreased incidence of intestinal disease including diverticular diseases (outpouchings in the intestine which become inflamed),

and possibly appendicitis, irritable bowel syndrome (alternating bouts of constipation and diarrhea), and cancer of the colon.

Exercise is another form of "nature's laxatives," because it stimulates the digestive system and tones the muscles therein for better efficiency. Ample fluid intake, too, aids nature in "regulating" the body. Therefore, instead of curtailing your father-in-law's diet, expand it fiberously—and get him really "moving" by buying him a good pair of walking shoes!

Ever since I reached adulthood, I found drinking milk causes gastric upset: cramps, bloating, gas and diarrhea. Isn't milk meant for adults to enjoy, too?

Many adults (and some children) have difficulty in digesting lactose, the sugar found in milk. To digest lactose, the enzyme called lactase is required; if it is unavailable or is not present in the gastrointestinal system in adequate amounts, lactose is not digested properly, but passes into the large intestine where it is fermented. Fermentation of the sugar causes the "gas", which in turn leads to discomfort and bloating. Diarrhea may be the unpleasant end result.

Fortunately, you may be able to gradually increase your tolerance to milk. Simply start small, perhaps several sips of milk a day, and gradually increase your intake to a full cup—perhaps split into smaller serving sizes at two or more meals. It is best to consult your physician before attempting this procedure, however, especially if your milk intolerance causes severe side effects. Many people who are unable to tolerate milk can enjoy fermented milk in the form of yogurt or kefir. Some can tolerate cheese. And for those who need them, there are lactose-reduced milk and special products which can be added to milk to digest the lactose before consumption. If all else fails, ask your physician about this. After all, one need not give up the pleasures of drinking milk along with the other enjoyments of youth.

Will lack of milk intake during the adult years lead to brittle bones in the later years?

Yes, it may do just that. "Brittle bones" or the disease known as osteoporosis, is a common affliction in the aging. In order to prevent or slow down the development of osteoporosis, calcium, vitamin D, and fluoride are all important dietary factors. Drinking an adequate amount of (calcium-rich) milk fortified with vitamin D and water fortified with the mineral nutrient fluoride is essential. If you cannot tolerate milk and if your water supply is not fluoridated, your physician may prescribe the appropriate supplements.

A non-dietary factor in the development of osteoporosis is lack of physical activity. Exercise builds stronger bones which are less apt to become brittle and fragile with age. Therefore, it is important for you to be physically active for as long as possible, in order to stay young from top to toe. Research indicates that osteoporosis may be associated less with the aging process itself and more with the decreased levels of physical activity which typically accompany an advance in years. So, drink your milk, get plenty of fresh air and exercise—sounds like what you may have told your children, grandchildren, and great-grand-children!

Is osteoporosis different from osteoarthritis? And is osteoarthritis the same as regular old, age-onset arthritis?

Osteoporosis is due to diminished bone density causing the bones to become porous, brittle and easily fractured; osteoarthritis is one of the many forms of the overall condition known as arthritis. Arthritis is not a single disorder, but an umbrella term which encompasses over 100 conditions of joint inflammation, including degenerative or osteo-arthritis, rheumatoid arthritis, and gout. Although arthritis is often considered a disease of old age, some forms affect children and young adults, while the various disorders are not an inevitable aspect of the aging process.

Affecting over 30 million Americans, arthritic conditions cause pain and inflammation around the joints and in the surrounding tissues. There is no known cure, but certain medications can help to relieve the pain and decrease the inflammation. Because the symptoms come and go, victims of arthritis often attribute "cures" to whatever occurred before the pain subsided. Often, dietary "miracle cures" are ac-claimed—until the symptoms reappear. Unfortunately, there has yet to be discovered an effective dietary cure for arthritis. Prevention measures include maintenance of general good health, a well-balanced diet, and a regular program of physical activity. Treatment includes the same measures along with prescribed medication and physical/ occupational therapy. Special adaptive equipment may be used, including helpful eating utensils.

Osteoarthritis tends to run in families, often affecting the small joints of the hands. Although the cause is unknown, some contributing causes to arthritis include overweight, injury, stress and strain, and heredity.

Avoid the temptation to purchase anti-arthritis "miracle" aids. As with most degenerative diseases, such claims appeal to your emotional hopes and fears, but the associated products can do little to actually prevent or treat the condition. Like cancer, those suffering from arthritis have long been prime targets for health quacks and pseudo-medical charlatans. Caveat emptor!

Then are all those advertisements for nutritional supplements for the elderly misleading? Don't I need Geritol for my iron-poor blood?

Unfortunately, most of the clamor over nutrition supplements—for individuals of all ages—is made by the companies promoting the products, the retailer who sells them, and the food faddists who mistakenly believe in the need for self-prescribed vitamins, minerals, and other unnecessary drugs (in large doses, even "natural" nutrients can be considered medicinal). Unless your physician has prescribed such supplementation due to a diagnosed deficiency, you should be getting all the nutrition you need at the kitchen table.

Nutritional anemias are not uncommon in older Americans, especially those subsisting on a low income. Although iron-deficiency anemia is the most common disorder, deficiencies in other nutrients can lead to the medical ailments which signal this disorder: a low intake of folic acid, sometimes noted in non-fruit-and-vegetable-favoring older populations, can cause anemia, as can the inadequate absorption of vitamin B_{12}, from which oldsters may suffer when their gastric juices become less ample.

However, unless a deficiency of iron or other nutrients has been determined by your physician, Geritol or any other self-prescribed nutrition supplement is probably not the key to the vim and vigor which all the advertisements seem to indicate. A far wiser, less costly, and more effective method to supply yourself with added energy is to engage in daily physical activity (see Chapter 3), adhere to a well-balanced diet with adequate calories selected from the Basic Four Food Groups (see Chapters 1 and 2), and keep busy with social activities, favorite hobbies, and good old-fashioned fun!

CHRONIC DISORDERS AFFECTED BY NUTRITION

My mother has been excessively fatigued lately, and even though she has been eating, has lost some weight. Diabetes runs in the family, but wouldn't she have gotten it before now, at least before she turned 65?

With this disease in the family, chances are good that adult-onset diabetes would afflict your mother before age 65—and may be a problem for you in the near future. In most cases, however, age is not the culprit but body weight is. If your mother has lost weight, this may be to her benefit if she is overweight. In fact, therapy for adult-onset diabetes includes diet for weight reduction to attain and maintain a reasonable weight.

Since you do suspect diabetes, have your mother visit the family physician for proper diagnosis. If this is indeed the case, your mother will be counseled about the appropriate diet for her to follow, and she may require medication (insulin injections or oral agents); and physical activity on a regular basis may be advised. Diabetes can be a startling discovery, but need not be an incapacitating disease. For the majority of adults who discover that they are diabetic, weight loss to a reasonable body weight and adherence to a well-balanced diet are all that is required to keep the disease under control.

It may be advisable for you, too, to reduce your weight to a reasonable level if necessary, and to follow a well-balanced diet plan like the ones outlined in this book. Prevention is preferable to treatment, and in adhering to a sensible program of diet and exercise, you may reduce your chances of ever developing diabetes—and other diseases as well.

My husband is recovering from a heart attack, his second since he turned 55. Should he try the Pritikin Diet to avoid another?

If your husband has had several heart attacks, chances are good that he has more than one of the following "risk factors" for heart disease: family history of heart disease at an early age (before 65); family history of diabetes; overweight; high blood pressure (hypertension); elevated blood cholesterol levels; history of cigarette smoking; physical inactivity; and a stressful lifestyle with a good deal of tension and anxiety.

Therefore, diet is only one factor which may have contributed to his heart condition. Yet, it is an important risk factor, one over which—unlike heredity—he can exert control.

The Pritikin Diet is an extremely restrictive plan which is limited in protein, marginal in sodium and fat, and eliminates many items from the diet such as caffeine, alcohol, and sugar. Nutritional deficiencies are a possibility on this diet for those who are able to adhere to it for any length of time (see Fad Diet chart in Chapter 2). The best aspect of the Pritikin plan, developed by a former heart disease patient without any medical or nutrition degrees, is the emphasis on daily exercise.

The American Heart Association (AHA) advocates a "prudent" diet for the treatment and possibly the prevention of heart disease. More liberal than the Pritikin regime, the AHA diet is similar to the sensible well-balanced diet described in this book, with total fat intake kept to 30 to 35% of total calories, a daily cholesterol intake below 300 milligrams (mg). Since there are around 250 mg of cholesterol in one egg, our most common source of this substance, the AHA diet limits egg consumption to 2 to 3 yolks per week, as well as moderation in sodium. A far more realistic and practical plan, almost anyone can follow a prudent diet such as the AHA's without nutritional threat or emotional deprivation.

The wisest step for your husband to take is to confer with his physician regarding the appropriate diet. Referral to a registered dietitian for professional individualized diet counseling may be advised. In this case, you should attend these counseling visits for menu assistance and diet tips from which both you and your husband can benefit.

If vegetarianism isn't the answer to a healthy heart, could it then be the route to a cancer-free future?

As with heart disease, vegetarians tend to have a better track record than non-vegetarians with certain cancers including breast, uterus, prostate, and colon. Although research is still under way, preliminary findings indicate that the low-fat, high-fruit/vegetable/grain diet may be protective against cancer. There are other factors of importance as well, including the tendency for vegetarians to avoid cigarette smoking, alcohol abuse, and perhaps stressful lifestyles as well.

Unfortunately, it is still too early to be able to determine just how much of a role diet plays in cancer prevention. Yet many claims are being made that specific diets can prevent or even cure this unpredictable disease. Be wary of undocumented pitches for special diets to ward off cancer, because such claims appeal to emotional, hope-filled human nature and ignore scientific fact. Often these diet plans include purchasing something to enrich the coffers of the diet's proponents; sometimes these diets are dangerous.

For example, Michio Kushi, founder of the macrobiotic diet movement in this country and vociferous proponent of "natural" foods, has recently published a book misleadingly entitled THE CANCER PREVENTION DIET: Blueprint for Relief and Prevention of Disease. Kushi's 460-page book is based on his own theory that the macrobiotic diet is the key to the prevention and cure of degenerative disease, including cancer. The macrobiotic diet is a strict vegetarian diet which permits no meat, poultry, eggs or milk products but includes an occasional serving of white-meat fish or seafood. Fruit is limited to once or twice weekly and is to be eaten cooked or dried. Tropical and semi-tropical fruits are taboo, including oranges, grapefruit and bananas. The other blackballed items are too numerous to list but include all common sweeteners, most vegetable oils, potatoes and tomatoes, and "all industrially mass-produced foods."

Will a vegetarian diet help us older folks ward off heart disease?

Although vegetarians do tend to have less incidence of heart disease, the meatless diet is no guarantee that heart health—and overall well-being—is optimized. The other risk factors for heart disease are important as well.

However, by eliminating meat from the diet, fat and cholesterol intake can be reduced significantly. If low-fat dairy products are used, along with an occasional egg, the vegetarian diet may be a healthful, nutritious one—as long as it includes generous servings from the Fruit and Vegetable Group, Bread and Cereal Group, as well as alternate sources of protein such as legumes and cottage cheese. Restrictive vegetarian diets which exclude all animal products including milk, cheese, and eggs are nutritionally unbalanced and may lead to deficiencies in iron, protein, calcium, vitamin B_{12}, and certain other nutrients. Don't short-change yourself nutritionally in search of a healthy diet plan!

The book's main danger lies in the prescriptive style enmeshed in a web of diet-cancer misinformation. The Cancer Prevention (i.e., macrobiotic) Diet is described while adoption is "supported" by "prophetic voices"—historical accounts of ancient provegetarians and deceptive statements of "research" summaries—including the National Academy of Science's diet-cancer report, misleadingly defined as "similar in direction" to macrobiotics. To state that "hundreds of thousands of people now following the Cancer Prevention Diet are free of worry from cancer, heart disease, and other degenerative illnesses" is an appetizing ploy for naive readers who want to be able to control their own destinies. It is also cruel to broadly inform all cancer patients that "he or she was directly responsible for the development of the disease."

Kushi appears not adverse to practicing medicine without a license. He advises cancer patients not to "combine the Cancer Prevention Diet with radiation or chemotherapy." And terminal cancer patients subscribing to macrobiotics are advised that they are more likely to recover than are those who have received conventional treatment. Drugs, including insulin, anticonvulsives, and blood pressure medications, are to be weaned away. Disappearance of pain is promised within ten days of dietary adoption. And even those without cancer are led to believe that "as many as 80 to 90 percent of modern people have some type of precancerous condition" including freckles, dry skin, and sinus problems!

At one point in the book, Kushi advises readers to "use common sense." Unfortunately, many cancer victims and a significant number of those prone to cancerphobia discard common sense in favor of misleading promises and magical cure-alls. The end results of the dangerous persuasions of such books often prove tragic.

Diet may play a role in the development of cancer (such as cancer of the colon), but there are a number of other factors to consider as well.

Thus, the vegetarian diet, macrobiotic regime, or other such eating patterns cannot guarantee you a cancer-free future. Diet is a way of living, not a religion in which to concentrate all of your faith and hopes.

My mother has terminal cancer and has lost a good deal of weight. She is bedridden, but not hospitalized. How can I help her to enjoy her last weeks, at least from a dietary standpoint?

The best advice is to do just as you plan, that is, to help her to enjoy her final weeks of life. By avoiding force-feeding and presenting her with attractive trays of appealing foods, you can help to make her days more comfortable.

We recommend *The Joy of Eating*, a brochure for cancer patients and their families (5413 Avenida Fiesta, La Jolla, CA, 92037; 1981). This helpful booklet includes sample menus, tips on nutritional problems, and other ideas for dealing with dietary dilemmas during cancer treatment. Author Jill Seagren, a registered dietitian, offers the following tips for stimulating appetite—perhaps some of her ideas can assist you in seeing that your mother is well fed.

STIMULATING THE APPETITE

- Keep high protein, or high calorie snacks which require little or no preparation in the house. When you feel like eating, nibble on these.
- Try eating frequent small portions, for example, a snack or small meal every other hour rather than three meals per day.
- Establish a set pattern of eating with meals and snacks at definite times. Stick to this schedule even when your appetite has deserted you.
- Eat with friends or family whenever possible.
- Make your food appetizing. A variety of colors and textures of food served attractively often stimulate a failing appetite.
- Sip on fluids that give you energy (juices, fruit drinks, milk, or even tea with sugar). Don't fill up on water, use your thirst to help you eat.
- Leave dishes of high calorie foods such as nuts, dried fruits and candy next to your bed or easy chair.
- Gentle exercise, for example a walk, before meals will often stimulate hunger.
- Leave snacks all over the house.
- Try a glass of beer or wine before your meals.
- Take pain or bowel medication one hour before eating so that its effect is maximal when you need it. (Check with the doctor about the timing of medications.)
- Strictly schedule yourself to eat a small quantity of food, for example, one bite, each hour of the day.

WHAT TO DO WHEN FOOD TASTES BAD
OR HAS NO TASTE

- Pleasant smells may help, for example, freshly baked bread, frying bacon, and simmering soup.
- If the taste of familiar food has changed or decreased, try eating warm foods with stimulating aromas.
- Very sweet foods often become unappealing. Avoid using sugar or sweeteners in recipes at this time.
- Tastebuds may become more sensitive; avoid highly seasoned or salty foods.
- If meat tastes bad, choose other high protein foods such as cheese, nuts, beans, or milk.
- Moist or liquid foods may taste better and be easier to swallow.
- Fruit nectars may be more palatable than fruit juices.
- Take a drink of liquid with each bite of food.
- Snack on popsicles, ice cream, or sherbets.
- Sometimes brushing your teeth before eating will help.
- Mildly acid foods, such as lemonade, may stimulate your taste-buds.
- Rely on other senses to provide some of the pleasure that flavor used to provide; for example, eat at a colorful place-setting, which includes flowers and candles. Eat foods of many colors and textures. Make your meals as appetizing to your eye as they were before to your taste.
- If you are restricted to liquid foods, try mixing a bland liquid formula with a sweet one, for example, tube feeding formula mixed with a flavored supplement like eggnog or instant breakfast drink to provide a nourishing, yet good-tasting food.

My uncle is in a well-run nursing home, but every time I visit him, he seems to have developed a new bedsore. If it isn't the nursing care, could his diet be causing this problem?

One million elderly citizens are in long-term care institutions or "nursing homes," which is around 5% of the over-65 population. One of the leading causes of death in the elderly is infection, and since undernutrition can cause increased susceptibility, proper diet is essential. Even though malnutrition per se is not often listed as the cause of death for the aged, poor diet is quite often a contributing factor to mortality in those getting along in years.

Bedsores, or "decubitus ulcers" as they are called in medical lingo, occur more frequently in overweight, underweight, and immobilized individuals. Thus, if your uncle is too heavy, too lean, or bedridden, the nursing staff should take heed and make the appropriate corrective changes. Also, anemia can worsen the condition, so you may want to ask about his most recent blood analysis. Dehydration affects bedsores, too, so the nursing staff should make sure that he gets plenty of fluids.

If it is indeed a reliable institution, your uncle's problem should be resolvable. However, improper care and poor attention to patients—more so than diet—can determine the comfort and longevity of your uncle's stay.

Are there any special dietary alterations to aid those with Parkinson's disease?

Parkinson's disease is a chronic neurological (nervous system) disorder characterized by gradually spreading tremor, muscular weakness and rigidity. Although the most common nervous disorder in older Americans (1% of those over age 50 are afflicted), the cause is unknown and recovery is rare. This disease usually appears during middle-age, but the older population are not immune. Victims of Parkinson's disease may require special dietary/feeding aids because of tremors and lack of coordination. Those taking levodopa need to avoid foodstuffs high in vitamin B_6 which interferes with the drug's action; the following is a list of foods to avoid: avocado, bacon, beans (legumes), beef liver, bread enriched with vitamin B_6, breakfast cereal enriched with vitamin B_6, bran enriched with vitamin B_6, kidneys, milk (whole, dry, and skim), nuts, peas, pork, salmon-fresh, tuna, wheat germ, yams, and yeast.

As with other degenerative diseases, undernutrition/weight loss needs to be prevented with appealing foods divided into 4 to 6 small meals and snacks, plus supplementation as necessary. Watch out for pseudo-nutrition hype claiming dietary "cures" and other pitches based on false hope (victim's) and pursuit of economic gain (supplement salesperson's). Physical activity appears to be helpful, and staying active mentally and socially can lessen the rate of decline as well.

Does improper diet cause Alzheimer's disease? I recently read that using aluminum in baking can cause the brain damage of this dreaded kind of premature senility.

Alzheimer's disease is due to gradual changes in the outer layer of the brain causing alterations in personality and function, including depression, moodiness, irritability, inability to perform routine tasks, reduced attention span, speech impediment, memory loss, and eventually poor self-care. The most common cause of intellectual impairment in the elderly population, about 6% of those over age 65 suffer from the severe form of premature senility (which actually includes a number of changes in the brain quite different from those of senility and aging). The cause and cure for Alzheimer's disease are as yet unknown.

Since 10% of those over age 65 suffer from brain disorders which affect normal functioning, this leaves 90% with no signs of mental impairment. Thus, the stereotype of senile aging individuals should be disregarded, and any symptoms such as forgetfulness and memory lapses, confusion, or hallucinations require immediate medical attention. For many, these problems can be reversed once the causes are identified.

As far as the aluminum–Alzheimer's relationship is concerned, there is not enough evidence to incriminate this common metal in the disease. Research is underway because certain studies have indicated that victims of the disease may have higher concentrations of aluminum in their brain cells. However, there is no proof of cause and effect, and certainly not enough reason to fear aluminum foil! Fortunately, research on Alzheimer's disease has increased over 500% since 1976. (For more information, write to the Alzheimer's Disease and Related Disorders Association, 360 No. Michigan Ave., Chicago, IL, 60601).

"PRESCRIPTION FOR SENILITY"

Can proper diet prevent the onset of senility?

Yes and No. Irreversible senility can be due to small strokes which reduce the blood supply to the brain, causing the mental confusion, disorientation and memory losses. The incidence of strokes can be reduced with control of blood pressure which, as you know, can be enhanced somewhat with proper diet. Reversible senility, however, can be due to the mental consequences of poor diet, drug use, or lack of stimulation. Such psychological disorders can be erased with a well-balanced diet, attention to drug use, and psychosocial interaction to prevent isolation and depression.

Memory loss is *not* a normal process of aging. Senility is a disease. Without illness, memory function and the ability for clear thinking do not lessen much with age. If untreated, so-called "senility" can lead to permanent disability requiring long-term care. With attention to diet and both physical and emotional needs, however, the reversible form of "senility" can be prevented, reversed, or at least lessened in severity.

Often attributed to or confused with senility, depression may be the cause or result of physical illness. Major life changes within brief time periods (e.g., loss of a spouse, change in residence, retirement, etc.) can trigger the onset of depression, ill health, and even death. Suicide stemming from severe depression occurs at a significant rate in the older population, and is especially prevalent in aged men.

Depression can lead to loss of appetite and weight, as well as to improper dietary habits and malnutrition. Nutritional deficiencies can then worsen the depression and contribute to the confusion, disorientation, and loss of memory diagnosed as senility. Insomnia, behavioral disorders ranging from apathy to psychoses, and alcoholism may develop, furthering the malnutrition and the deteriorating state of mental health.

Depressed individuals may turn to overeating in search of emotional support. Food can temporarily act to relieve anxiety and diminish loneliness. Often, the overabundant dietary intake is based on high-fat, high-calorie foodstuffs and excludes the more preferable, nutrient-rich items. Thus, the depressed overeater may be building up certain nutrient deficiencies along with unwanted body fat. Arthritis, diabetes, heart disease, and other health disorders associated with obesity can only act to worsen the depression.

"Senility" can afflict you before you even have a chance to enter into your "golden years." The disorder and its vague symptoms may spiral, due to organic and/or functional causes which intensify the severity of the problem. Early intervention with required medical treatment, psychological counseling, and nutritional management can mean the difference between debilitating depression and the mental clarity which can illuminate your "golden years."

Watch out for diet fads which claim to markedly improve memory, for such promotions are money-making schemes to sell useless supplements. Such purchases are always a waste of money, and may cause nutritional imbalances as well. You are better off to "forget" about such rip-offs, and "remember" instead to eat a well-balanced diet and to exercise regularly.

What side effects can drugs cause besides "senility"? So many of us older adults have to take medication.

Comprising only about 10% of the population, the elderly now account for nearly one-quarter of the drugs that are prescribed and the over-the-counter medications that are in use. An estimated 85% of the aged use prescription drugs, and the typical older individual fills more than a dozen prescriptions each year. As an average senior citizen, you could expect to spend at least $100 this year on drugs, more than you would spend at any other time in your life.

Unfortunately, age makes you more susceptible to the undesirable side effects of drug use. If you are poorly nourished during your later years, you may suffer even more from potential side effects (including drug-drug and food-drug interactions) as the aging body becomes less capable of handling drugs and nutrients properly. The absorption, distribution, metabolism, and/or excretion of drugs and nutrients may be altered in the aged body, and certain conditions such as underweight, dehydration, and low protein intakes can exaggerate drug strength. Therefore, as you grow older, it is imperative that you exercise more care in the use of both prescription and over-the-counter drugs, and that you become aware of any nutritional implications.

Should I discontinue taking these medications, then? Maybe I can just be sure to follow a healthy diet instead.

Diet must be viewed realistically: Although it plays an important role in overall health, diet is not the cause nor the cure of all ills. Therefore, dropping all other health aids with false hopes in dietary magic is like putting all your eggs in one basket—destined for a fall!

If you want to change or discontinue drug use, discuss this important change with your physician. Even with over-the-counter medications, it is important to talk to your doctor before you make any alterations. Using common sense in drug, diet, and health care is a plus in your favor.

SOCIAL ISSUES AFFECTING DIET

I'm so lonely, I think I have begun to go senile! I keep forgetting to eat, and am worried that my poor diet will ruin my health. Any tips for a thin, lonely widower?

Stimulation is the key to psychological and physical health—and to the avoidance of emotional confusion and nutritional depletion. If you are lonely and isolated, you may want to combine your need for dietary improvement with social contacts: Find out if there are congregate meal sites in your area where older citizens gather for a hot lunch and camaraderie; if you are house-bound, see if there is a Meals-on-Wheels or other food delivery program to provide nutrition and outside contact in the form of a daily meal delivery visit; join a food or meal co-op with other older "singles", or form your own dinner group to share in food preparation and in dining. You may want to refer to the next chapter for shopping, cooking, and preparation tips as well as recipe ideas.

With the growth in the older population, there is no need for you to be lonely. There are plenty of other "golden agers" in need of companionship, too. And many younger folks could undoubtedly benefit from your friendship—and perhaps your culinary skills—as well.

Ever since I turned 65 and was forced to retire, I have become increasingly isolated and depressed. Needless to say, my diet has suffered for it: TV-dinners every night are as boring as they are nutrition-less. How can I get out of this rut, at least as far as my diet is concerned?

TV-dinners are not nutrient-free, and some of the modern frozen dinners are high-nutrient, low-calorie, delicious-tasting meals. The major drawback nutritionally is that many are quite high in sodium. Read the labels to determine nutritional composition, and you may want to taste-test some of the newer choices before you prematurely condemn all such products.

As long as your diet is varied and well-balanced, there is room for frozen dinners on occasion. Just be sure to include adequate amounts of fruits, vegetables, whole grains and low-fat milk products, and to emphasize the leaner cuts of meat, fish and poultry. And if a diet of TV dinners means a lifestyle planted in front of the television set, you may want to incorporate more activity and less sedentary TV-viewing into your daily patterns. (The older population watches more television per day in general than any other age group!)

TV-dinners may not be the essential factor you need to consider, however, because the "rut" you are in is more important than the dietary boredom it has caused. If you are lonely and/or depressed, socializing can help to improve your emotional health as well as your diet. Entertaining guests, joining clubs and groups, occasionally dining out will help to get you out of that TV-rut. At any age, too much time in the role of armchair viewer is unhealthy, unstimulating, isolating, and unappetizing. Hopefully, you can push yourself out of the armchair and into all that society has to offer today's elder citizens motivated enough to seek stimulation.

My father is almost 100 years old! But he has been bedridden now for almost a year, and has begun to decline physically (not mentally, though!) including gradual weight loss. How can I entice him to keep up his strength, and are there effective methods for increasing his caloric intake in an appetizing manner?

At his age, your father is doing fantastically well, especially if his mental faculties are still sharp. If lack of appetite is the problem, you need to prepare appealing meals and snacks which are not over-whelming in size. It is essential that wasting and malnutrition be prevented, so special nutritional supplements might be helpful: "instant breakfasts" are tasty and nutritious, and there are a variety of other powdered and liquid formulas available in pharmacies. Ask your father's physician for suggestions. And congratulate your father for us for living to such a ripe old age!

My diet is dull and drab, mainly because my retirement benefits are "the pits," as they say these days. How can I eat well without spending a fortune?

It is essential to be a smart shopper these days, in order to stretch the food budget as far as possible. Some tips for accomplishing this are provided in the following chapter. However, if your benefits are inadequate to cover food bills, you may want to take advantage of the Food Stamp program.

The quantity of Food Stamps you are entitled to receive depends on your monthly household income. These stamps are purchased at reduced fees to be used like money for purchasing food (or plants/seeds, but not for buying inedible products), but cannot be sold or used to pay up old debts at the grocery store. Only those stores with signs indicating "We Accept Food Coupons" participate in the federally funded program. NOTE: Many individuals are too proud to seek aid. This program was developed to assist you, not to degrade you. Take advantage of the fact that you have long supported the government with your taxes, and it is time now for the government to help to support *you*.

Where else can I obtain information on benefits for older citizens?

The Food Stamp Program is administered through local welfare departments. Feeding programs for the elderly are provided under Title III (formerly Title VII) of the Older Americans Act; call your local hospital to find out where the congregate meals are held in your city or town, or to determine how to begin a home-delivery service. Home health services, including help with food shopping/preparation, are provided by public or private agencies for home-bound individuals upon physician referral. The RSVP (Retired Senior Volunteer Program) helps elder citizens both physically and socially, whereas other community programs can provide services and telephone/personal contact (e.g., Friendly Visitors, F.I.S.H., etc.). Your town's chamber of commerce can help you to identify the program which may be able to meet your needs. Public and church-related social service agencies may also be of assistance, and local senior citizen/retirement groups can provide additional support and social contact (see Appendix C for additional services and addresses).

Are there any places older citizens can contact when they think they have been "ripped off"? I purchased a nutrition supplement to "cure" my arthritis, and after spending a lot of money, there is absolutely no improvement. My elderly friends constantly complain of similar disappointments. With my meager income, I cannot afford to lose money this way. Any advice?

As you have learned, it is important for you to beware of phony health claims and diet-related rip-offs. You should report any such occurrence to the local Better Business Bureau, the Food and Drug Administration, and the Dietary Department of your local hospital, as well as alert your physician and your friends to the invalid claim. In your case, a letter to the Arthritis Foundation would be appropriate. The addresses for the national organizations are included in Appendix C. The key to wise health care expenditures is common sense: With a well-balanced diet based on the Basic Four Food Groups, plus an active lifestyle conducive to good health, you will lay the foundation for optimal well-being. And by avoiding fad diets and health gimmickry, you can build a long and healthy life while saving yourself from unnecessary expenditures and dashed hopes. Again, Caveat emptor!

Congressman Claude Pepper

An avid battler against the rampant health fraud which plagues today's older population, Congressman Claude Pepper expends much energy fighting for our right to be healthy. In order to maintain his own youthful vigor, Pepper ensures adequate energy by eating a hearty, well-balanced diet and expends some of that energy in brisk daily walks or by playing golf. His dietary and exercise patterns have not changed much during the past few (busy!) decades, except that he now opts for more seafood, chicken, or lean veal in place of beef or other high-fat red meats. A typical menu for the Chairman of the Senate Select Committee on Aging (aged 84) would consist of the following:

Breakfast	*Lunch*	*Dinner*
raisin bran cereal with skim milk and sliced banana	thick soup with crackers	thick soup with crackers
cheese toast	seafood sandwich	broiled fish, chicken, or veal
beverage	green salad with blue cheese dressing	potato, mashed
	pie	1 or 2 steamed vegetables
		tossed salad with blue cheese dressing
		ice cream

Once my minor ills are taken care of, my diet is balanced, and my body is physically fit, will I still feel old?

*How old is old? Old, by consensus the last phase of human life before death, has had different meanings, different numbers of years, and different realities throughout the history of the human family.

If we were living in antiquity, "old" was any time between the ages of 20 to 25; average life expectancy ranged between 8–20 years! By the Middle Ages, with the disappearance of Roman emphasis on sanitary conditions and bodily cleanliness, the average life expectancy decreased to 14. The Early Renaissance was marked by an improvement to the age of 20. During the 17th and 18th centuries the average life expectancy had moved to 25 and 30 years, followed by an increase to 47 years by the 19th century.

Today, in the ninth decade of the 20th century, that average in our society has reached 74.5 years (71 for men and 78 for women).

Is old what we see—the wrinkled skin, the gray hair, dull eyes, hesitant gait and stooped shoulders?

Is old the functional decline with the years—the decrease in metabolism, in failing cardiovascular efficiency, the loss of flexibility, speed and muscle strength, the changing EEG and sleep patterns, slower nerve conduction?

Is old the confused, forgetful, undecided, cantankerous over-65 who lives in the memories of the past, no longer interested in the present, facing a minimal, meaningless future?

Is old the socially isolated, obsolete, segregated non-worker, the roleless, soon to be invalidated burden, the asexual, unloving unlovable shadow of a former human being?

Is old the disease-ridden, dependent patient waiting eagerly for death as the only way to peace and freedom from pain?

Is old a natural state—all the accumulated changes with time that result in increased vulnerability to disease and death—genetically based, but environmentally modulated?

Or, is old often an imposed classification for those society wishes to defuse, to remove from full view, and to dehumanize?

Old may be characterized by a little, some, or all of these. Old may fit the stereotypes suggested, grown out of fear of the emptiness that has so long been carved by contemporary American civilization—fulfilling the expectations learned from childhood forward.

Although some older persons do succumb to the chronic diseases more prevalent in the later years, many do not. Though some elderly do withdraw from social activities, most want to remain integrated in the society. Though some are markedly less able, less vigorous, many are not. Aging is not disease—although vulnerability to dysfunction and disease increases with the years.

There is no magic about age 65. This is the birthday which has come to signify "old" in the U.S. today. This convention relates to the choice in 1932 of the then developing U.S. Social Security plan. Age 65 became the birthday of retirement.

---

*Reprinted with permission from *The Professional Nutritionist*, Winter, 1979, p. 3.

The work before (all of) us (young and old) includes not only the reduction of chronic diseases in incidence and severity with eventual prevention, not only the maintenance of vitality and motivation into the later years, but the drastic alteration of attitude toward aging and old. It is the current myopia of fear and ignorance about aging and old that makes it possible for this nation to still worship at the altar of youth—and to lose the resource that is the talent, experience, and the growing personality of the old.

We suggest that, in addition to adopting a healthy lifestyle as outlined in this book, those individuals who feel old should simply stop having birthdays. According to Dr. Robert Kastenbaum, geriatric specialist at the University of Massachusetts, the annual birthday celebration is actually adding to our wrinkles, since conscious awareness of the passage of time contributes to physical aging. Ignore your birthday, and you may find that you have more of them. On the other hand, you certainly won't receive many birthday presents, and you may miss the annual delicious cake and ice cream as well!

Mervyn LeRoy
(of Mervyn LeRoy Productions, age 84)

"I would not recommend my dietary practices or exercise program to anyone because I eat all the wrong things and don't exercise at all. Despite all this, I'm in pretty good health and I feel wonderful!"

Part V

Just Desserts: Planning Meals For One Or Two

Julia Child: Moderation in All Things

Julia Child does not look as if she is over 70 years of age, as she skillfully prepares gourmet dishes and guides her fans through complex recipes. Much of her "youth" appears attributable to her "joie de vivre," and part may be due to her sensible, healthful lifestyle.

Julia's daily diet consists of "good fresh food" and, although careful of her fat intake for weight control purposes, she admits that she "loves red meat, and have it 4–5 times a week." Julia describes a typical day's menu as follows (including a great tip for a light cocktail):

"Breakfast is fruits, tea, and plain toast; lunch is salad and/or soup and cheese of some sort (calcium!); dinner is meat/fish/poultry/pasta plus fresh vegetables and no dessert unless we have company. Wine always accompanies dinner. Wine is less fattening as an apéritif than hard liquor, unfortunately! A favorite apéritif is a 'reverse martini' with lots of dry white French vermouth on lots of ice in a wine glass, with a gin float and a lemon peel. But that is more fattening than a glass of wine, alas."

Perhaps Julia's overall lifestyle philosophy can serve as one last summary on health and longevity in the later years. Here is a sensible guide dictated by an amazing woman who sets such an inspirational example for all:

"My philosophy is moderation in all things: eat a great variety of foods, exercise as much as possible, learn to deal with stress and tension, have plenty of good work to do and good friends to be with, and pick your parents (long-lived, that is) carefully."

JUST DESSERTS: PLANNING MEALS FOR ONE OR TWO

Psychological and physical preparation for your later years should commence early in life. Those older persons who have remained lean, eaten well, and kept physically active are better equipped to handle the changes and stresses which occur with aging. Yet, even if you are fortunate enough to succeed in facing old age with a healthy body and a sharp mind, age-specific problems which can threaten your good health may arise.

Retirement is often equated with diminished usefulness and decreased respect. Loss of identity may occur with the end of an active career, death of a spouse, moving on of children and grandchildren, etc. Thus, old age brings about the need for new methods to achieve recognition and feelings of self-worth. Recent growth in elderly volunteer programs, Golden Age groups, senior citizens' rights, and educational opportunities for older individuals attest to societal change supportive of your psychosocial needs upon entering the "golden years."

When you reach the age of retirement, the environmental determinants of your physical and mental health can be varied, but will depend largely on your individual living situation: *institutionalization*–in hospital, extended care, or other fully dependent facility, *living alone*–with no dietary assistance provided, *living alone*–receiving dietary assistance either in the home or in a group setting, *living with family*–dependent on others for dietary assistance, *living with friends*–residing in a group home, retirement village, or other supportive setting which supplies dietary assistance.

Depending on your living situation, obtaining an adequate diet as an elderly individual can be quite difficult. If you are fortunate enough to be living in a physically comfortable and emotionally stimulating environment, your health and nutritional status should respond favorably. However, if you become a member of the significant proportion of the older population *not* well tended, the environmental effects on health and nutrition may prove to be devastating.

If you find yourself in an institutional setting at some point during your later years, it is important to realize that the food service department is responsible for providing you with nutritious meals in an atmosphere which encourages dining pleasure. Thus, if your physical and/or emotional needs are not being met, it becomes your responsibility to discuss serious complaints with the administrator(s), doctors, nursing staff, dietary department, or assigned social workers. Attentive relatives may also be of assistance in procuring dietary needs.

105

If you are living alone when entering your "golden years," you may also find that your physical and emotional needs are unfulfilled. Failing health and depression can be improved with outside assistance. Feeding programs such as Meals-on-Wheels provide elderly individuals with ready-made meals that meet nutritional needs and are home delivered. Mobile individuals can enjoy nutritious luncheons in congenial social settings by attending a local congregate feeding site; these programs are usually operated by volunteers to offer the elderly a hot meal in the company of their peers, and some also provide a few minutes of education on a topic of interest such as food budgeting or health concerns. Such community programs typically provide a single daily meal which meets one-third of their RDA's; sometimes a brown bag with a sandwich, fruit, and milk is also supplied to be eaten later in the day. In either case, participants are still responsible for obtaining the remainder of their own individual daily dietary needs.

In Chicago, over 6,000 elder citizens meet at noontime on weekdays in over 100 sites to enjoy a hot meal as part of the federally funded "Golden Diners' Club." Menus vary, depending on the ethnic trends in the area: Chinese, Spanish, American Indian, Italian, Filipino, Puerto Rican, "soul", and kosher menus are served along with all-American fare in a variety of attractive, nutritious forms. And in Milwaukee, oldsters and youngsters dine together on hot lunches, because the majority of the city's public schools are open to elder citizens for discount noontime meals.

Another alternative for improving the diet is for older individuals to form or join food co-ops or cooking groups. If a number of your associates or neighbors band together, you can tackle together the problem of buying, preparing, and eating good food at affordable prices. Or you may have a friend or two who will trade-off on cooking meals, so that you can share recipes and dine together in addition to cutting down on food wastes and expenditures. You may even incorporate nutrition information into your own group meals by discussing the diet information you obtain (from reputable sources, of course) and sharing nutrition books (such as this one). Such group interaction should serve to improve your social life as well as your dietary intake.

MENU PLANNING TIPS

Is there an easy method to ensure that one's diet will be well-balanced every day without having to hire a personal nutritionist to review daily menu plans?

Fortunately, you need not employ a dietitian to scrutinize your food intake, nor need you be overly concerned about your diet to the point of stress and unreasonable anxiety. As outlined in the first chapter, a sensible diet can be followed quite easily and food heartily enjoyed. You only need to be sure to include a wide variety of foods in moderate amounts which are selected from the Basic Four Food Groups. If you include plenty of fruits and vegetables—especially citrus and dark green/deep yellow produce—breads, cereals, pastas and grain foods, as well as several daily servings of low-fat milk and its products, and lean meats, poultry, fish, plus occasional legumes, cottage cheese, and eggs, in amounts which allow you to attain and maintain a reasonable weight, few nutritionists could find fault with your diet.

As for menu planning, it is a matter of practicing by doing: if you make out a new menu at the beginning of each week which is well-balanced and meets your individual needs and desires, it should not prove difficult to follow. As situations arise, substitutions may need to be made. That's okay—be flexible, it will probably be more exciting. Vary your menus from day-to-day and week-to-week. Take heed of seasonal foods, holiday specials, and new products. With time, you may enjoy the act of devising creative menus almost as much as you look forward to eating the meals you have planned!

Could you provide some sample menus for a week of well-balanced meals for a retired couple (with hearty appetites and adventurous tastes)?

It's good to know that retirement has spiced up your appetites . . . for food—and living. Let's hope that you are retired *only* from your previous place of employment, but not from life's many opportunities and excitements. Now that you no longer have to spend a good portion of your time at work, you have more freedom and flexibility to enjoy your expanded leisure time. Eating can become a recreation providing much pleasure, menu planning a creative activity, and cooking a new (or improved) hobby.

The following menu plan includes a week of well-balanced meals, some samples for you to examine. Since your own individual needs and desires—and those of your spouse—should be met by the meals you eat, this menu can only serve as a guide to assist you in devising your own plan. After all, if you hate liver and love beer, there is no sense in adhering to a menu which includes the former and excludes the latter!

NOTE: The meals are given in serving sizes for one, and are relatively low in calories; these samples may be calorically inadequate if you are physically active, so plan your own menus and adjust portion size accordingly.

Day One

Breakfast:

1/2 grapefruit
1 sl. whole wheat toast with

Lunch:

sandwich: 2 sl. rye bread broiled with
1 oz. part-skim mozzarella cheese and

1 tsp. peanut butter and
1/2 banana, sliced
1 cup skim milk

Dinner:

3 oz. lean roast veal
1/2 cup applesauce
1 cup wax beans
tossed salad with French dressing
dinner roll
fig bar

sliced mushrooms, tomato
1/2 cup fruit cocktail

Snack:

1 cup yogurt, low-fat with
1/2 cup strawberries

Day Two

Breakfast:

1/2 cup orange juice
1 sl. raisin toast with
1 egg, scrambled with
1/4 cup cottage cheese, low-fat, and
    chives

Lunch:

spinach salad: fresh spinach with
sliced mushrooms, tomatoes, and
    croutons (toasted herbed French
    bread); plus
Italian dressing
fresh peach

Dinner:

1/2 cup spaghetti with
1 cup cooked tomato and
2 T grated parmesan cheese
tossed salad with oil and vinegar
1 sl. angel food cake with
1/4 cup fresh strawberries

Snack:

2 graham crackers
1 cup skim milk

Day Three

Breakfast:

1/4 cup prune juice
1 sl. rye toast
1 cup hot wheat cereal with
1/2 cup skim milk and
2 T raisins

Lunch:

sandwich: 1 sl. oatmeal bread with
1 T peanut butter and
1/2 tsp. honey
fresh orange

Dinner:

4 oz. dry chablis wine
chicken "cordon bleu": 3 oz. chicken
    baked with
1 oz. part-skim mozzarella cheese and
sliced mushrooms
1 cup spinach
tossed salad with French dressing
1 cup fruit salad

Snack:

date bar
1 cup skim milk

Day Four

Breakfast:

1/2 cup grapefruit juice
English muffin with
1 oz. low-fat cheese, melted

Lunch:

chef's salad: lettuce, assorted
    vegies, and
1 oz. sliced chicken and
1 oz. farmer's cheese plus
Greek dressing
breadsticks
1/2 cup applesauce

Dinner:

3 oz. lean hamburger on roll with
lettuce, sliced tomato and
1 oz. part-skim mozzarella cheese
1/2 cup baked beans
1 cup melon balls

Snack:

bran muffin, with
1 tsp. margarine
1 cup skim milk

Day Five

Breakfast:

1 cup fruit salad
1 egg, poached on
1 sl. oatmeal bread with
1 oz. mozzarella cheese, melted

Lunch:

sandwich: 2 sl. rye bread with
2 oz. sliced turkey and
1 tsp. mayonnaise and
lettuce, tomato
fresh pear

Dinner:

spinach-noodle bake:
1/2 cup spinach noodles with
1/4 cup cottage cheese, low-fat, and
1 cup chopped tomatoes, plus
sliced mushrooms, seasonings
tossed salad with oil and vinegar
baked peach half with
1/2 tsp. honey
1 cup skim milk

Snack:

12 oz. "light" beer
3–4 pretzel rings

Day Six

Breakfast:

1/2 cantaloupe (5" dia.) filled with
1/4 cup cottage cheese, low-fat
1 biscuit shredded wheat with
1/2 cup skim milk

Lunch:

1 sl. pumpernickel, topped and
    broiled with
1/2 cup cottage cheese, low-fat, with
chives and chopped mushrooms,
    garlic, herbs
fresh tangerine

Dinner:

1 cup Chinese-style assorted veggies,
  stir-fried with
1 oz. chopped chicken and
2 T peanuts on
1/2 cup brown rice
1 cup skim milk

Snack:

3 cups popcorn with
2 T parmesan cheese

Day Seven

Breakfast:

2–3 dried prunes
whole wheat bagel with
1 oz. part-skim mozzarella cheese,
  melted
1 cup skim milk

Lunch:

1 sl. raisin bread with
1/4 cup cottage cheese, low-fat, and
1/2 cup crushed pineapple
carrot sticks

Dinner:

4 oz. dry wine
4 oz. broiled halibut with lemon
1 cup broccoli, cauliflower, brussels
  sprouts medley
tossed salad with Italian dressing
baked potato, med., with low-fat
  yogurt and chives

Snack:

1/2 cup ice milk or frozen yogurt with
1/2 cup fresh strawberries

Additional Menu Notes

Meats should be lean, trimmed, and prepared without added fats by baking, boiling, broiling, or roasting. Poultry should have the skin removed and be prepared without added fats by baking, boiling, broiling, or roasting. Fish should be prepared (with minimal addition of margarine) by baking, boiling, broiling, or poaching; canned fish should be the water-packed varieties. Yogurt should be made with low-fat milk. Cheeses should be made with part-skim or skim milk. Fruit should be fresh, frozen, or canned without heavy syrups. Vegetables should be fresh or frozen without added sauces. Grains (breads, cereals, pastas, rice) should be 100% whole grain or enriched; if constipation is a problem, include bran-containing cereals often. Salad dressings should be the low-fat, low-calorie varieties. Prepare popcorn in hot-air popper to avoid use of oil. If you add margarine to toast, potato, or rolls, do so sparingly. Non-caloric beverages can be included as desired—coffee, tea, decaffeinated drinks, water, mineral water, club soda, iced tea, diet soft drinks—but moderation is always wise.

By following the menus I prepare in advance, food shopping is much easier and I only need to go once a week. Are there any tips for being a smart supermarket shopper?

If you only like to shop once a week, and find this practice to be practical when you utilize prepared menu plans, then the tips listed below may help to ease your food shopping burden and reduce the associated costs. However, some people find that more frequent food shopping trips are preferable, even daily expeditions. For these folks, an excuse to get out of the house or the apartment, a nice stroll in the fresh air, the chance to chat with neighbors, supermarket personnel and even to make new friends are practical reasons to regard food shopping as more than just a method to fulfill menu planning needs.

There are some definite drawbacks, however, to frequent shopping ventures for those in their later years. Shopping can prove to be quite a challenge due to transportation problems; travel routes to and from plus the demographics of area shopping centers; difficulties in toting groceries; inclement weather; and the general confusion which can erupt during a stressful event. If you are unable to drive or have difficulties walking and carrying bundles, just getting to the store and back may be impossible. Busy streets, dangerous neighborhoods, poor sidewalks, and inaccessible supermarket layouts can add to your difficulties. If the winter cold poses a problem with being outdoors, the intense heat of the summer is not much easier for going shopping, even if lugging heavy loads is not too difficult for you.

Some supermarkets make available senior citizen buses. In certain cities and towns, volunteer organizations provide transport for the elderly. If poor health or other problems interfere with your ability to shop for food, you may want to find out if such services are available, especially if you live alone and do not wish to impose on friends or neighbors.

The choice of a supermarket which can meet your needs should take your individual lifestyle into consideration: the post-war boom in shopping centers has led to a surge in supermarket chains which offer a large variety of foodstuffs including fresh produce and the latest products, as well as customer services. Unfortunately, these large chains are geared to the able-bodied, independent, and financially well-to-do shopper, but may not be practical for those with very low incomes or in ill health. The smaller neighborhood groceries often will deliver, accept phone orders, and may even maintain a running bill.

Thus, the supermarket(s) appropriate for your current needs should be selected carefully from those available in your city or town.

TIPS FOR SMART SUPERMARKET SHOPPING

- Plan menus in advance.
- Make a shopping list.
- Check newspapers for "specials" and use coupons for items that are on your list and a good buy.
- Follow your shopping list without deviations, and avoid impulse shopping.
- Avoid supermarket enticements, end of aisle "sales", and point-of-purchase "buys".
- Avoid shopping when hungry.
- Read labels carefully to check for ingredients, serving size, nutrients, and caloric contents—note that label nutrition information does not give % RDA's for older adults.
- Try the generic and less known brands.
- If you have a freezer, buy meats on sale in quantity to rewrap and freeze in individual packages.
- Alternate sources of protein—cottage cheese, legumes, peanut butter, eggs—are often less expensive than meat.
- Grade B brown eggs are cheaper but nutritionally equivalent to Grade A white eggs.
- Day-old bread is usually a good buy.
- Make sure your supermarket is consumer-oriented.
- Ask for smaller packaging, if you want it, and use the deli department.
- It may prove less costly (due to reduced waste) to buy prepared foods versus ingredients in too-large quantities.
- Cereals in individual serving sizes are more expensive as are the instant hot cereals.
- Non-fat dried milk is less expensive, requires little storage concern, and can be used to extend regular milk and/or enhance the protein quality of recipes.
- Leaner cuts of meat supply more protein for your money; use leftovers in casseroles, salads, sandwiches, soups, and with vegetable dishes. Often the cheaper cuts are just as tasty as the more expensive meats—as long as the cook uses skill, a little tenderizer, and creativity in preparation (see E-Z ENTRÉES for some suggestions).
- Do not be too proud to use food stamps if you so qualify: better to be well-nourished at federal expense than ill at your own!

Cooking for one lacks excitement, thus my diet is equally drab. Are there any magic methods for livening up my monotonous menu?

Yes, fortunately there are many seemingly "magic" methods for transforming even the bleakest diet into a fun-filled exciting menu plan. How? First, make sure that your dining atmosphere is conducive to fine eating: use attractive place settings, put a nice centerpiece on the table or eat at the window with the best view, invite friends to join you, and—once in a while—dine out. (Lunching out at off hours can frequently provide you with a hot meal at reduced rates.)

Next, take the time and make the effort to try out new foods and test out new recipes: drab can become delicious overnight. Make your menus a challenge to your creative juices and your meals will be a pleasant sensation down to your digestive juices! You might want to borrow from your local library or purchase some of the cookbooks suggested in Appendix C. And several of our own favorite delicious, nutritious recipes have been provided below.

EASY RECIPE IDEAS

Breakfast Bonus—Fast But Fine

- Fix a bowl of fresh or canned fruit and top it with a scoop of low-fat cottage cheese or yogurt; sprinkle with nuts or seeds, or try some sweet banana chips on top.
- The following ready-to-eat cereals are high in fiber, so can make for a quick, nutritious breakfast when served with low-fat milk and fruit or fruit juice: All-Bran, Bran Buds, 100% Bran, Most, Shredded Wheat, Wheaties, Total, and Grape-Nut Flakes; Wheatena, Ralston, Oatmeal, and Farina are hot cereal choices with favorable fiber contents. Mix several different kinds of cereals together to vary flavor and texture, and top with a sprinkling of the high-calorie kinds, such as granolas and Grape-Nuts.
- Slice a melon in half, scoop out the seeds, and fill with low-fat cottage cheese and berries in season.
- At the donut shop, order a bran muffin, juice, and low-fat milk.
- Roll wheat bread to flatten, spread with low-fat cottage cheese, top with cinnamon; roll up and bake at 350 degrees until bubbly; serve topped with canned peaches, pears, or other fruit.
- Fill a Syrian pocket with low-fat mozzarella cheese and bake at 350 degrees until cheese melts; serve with fruit juice.

Non-Breakfast Breakfasts

- Try a slice of carrot cake, or a piece of zucchini, pumpkin, or banana bread with a glass of low-fat milk.

- If they appeal, have a sandwich and/or soup (see Soups To Sup and Sandwiches To Savor).
- Leftovers often taste great first thing in the morning—hot or cold: pizza, casseroles, chicken, etc., washed down with fruit juice and/or low-fat milk.
- Hot low-fat milk drinks can help to perk you up, with or without caffeine: coffee, tea, or cereal beverages, such as Postum with milk, café au lait, Ovaltine or low-calorie Alba for hot chocolate, warm milk flavored with iron-rich molasses; add a slice of toast and a glass of juice for a well-balanced breakfast.

Recipes to Try

Light Granola—150 calories per ½ cup

2 cups rolled oats
1 cup wheat germ
1 cup wheat flakes cereal
½ cup non-fat dried milk
¼ cup raisins
2 tbsp. unsalted peanuts
1 tsp. cinnamon
1 tsp. vanilla
3/4 to 1 cup water

Mix dry ingredients. Add vanilla to water and mix into dry ingredients. Spread into a shallow baking pan and bake at 350 degrees for 15 minutes, then at 250 degrees, stirring occasionally, for 1–2 hours, until cereal appears dry. Makes 4 cups.

Homestyle Jam—20 calories per tbsp.

1 cup dried apples
1 cup dried peaches
1 cup dried pears
1 cup apple juice

Mix fruits with juice in saucepan, and simmer for 10 minutes until softened. Cool, use blender to purée, store in jars in refrigerator. Makes 4 cups.

Soups to Sup—Quickies*

- Heat up a can of your favorite soup and serve with wheat crackers and low-fat milk.
- The little boxes of individual servings of instant soup are rather expensive, but certainly convenient and fast.
- Heat up chicken, beef, or vegetable bouillon (cubes, canned, or powdered form) with leftover vegetables and rice.

---

*Canned and dried soups are high in sodium, but low-sodium varieties are available.

- Turn leftover vegetables into a cold gazpacho-type soup by chopping in the blender and spicing up with Italian herbs.
- Save water from cooked vegetables to use as the base or stock for homemade soups.
- Always make meat-based soups with cold water, since hot water seals the flavor into the meat.
- To freeze soup, chill overnight first, and remove fat from top. Be sure to leave room in container for expansion, and to label with content and date.

Recipes

Old Fashioned Vegetable Soup—75 calories

8 cups water or vegetable stock
2 carrots, chopped
1 onion, diced
1 cup celery, chopped
2 garlic cloves, minced
2 tbsp. basil
2 tbsp. parsley flakes
2 cups green beans
2 cups zucchini, diced
1 cup cooked white beans
1 cup corn niblets
1 cup tomato, diced
pepper

Combine liquid with carrots, onion, celery, garlic, basil, and parsley in large pot and bring to a boil. Simmer for 30 minutes. Add next 3 vegetables and simmer for 30 minutes more. Add corn and tomatoes, cook for 20 more minutes, and season with pepper. Makes 8 (1 cup) servings.

Black Bean Soup—125 calories

1 cup dried black beans
1 garlic clove, minced
1 sm. onion, chopped
4 cups water or vegetable stock
1 tbsp. oregano
2 tbsp. vinegar
hot pepper seasoning
low-fat yogurt, plain

Wash beans and soak overnight in 4 cups of cold water. In large pot, bring beans, bean water, garlic, onion, and water or stock to a boil, cover, and simmer for 1½ hours. Add seasonings and continue cooking for an hour or until beans are tender. Serve with a dollop of yogurt. Makes 6 (1 cup) servings.

Lentil Soup—195 calories

2 cups dried lentils
2 carrots, chopped

4 celery stalks, chopped
2 med. onions, diced
2 sm. potatoes, diced
2 garlic cloves, minced
2 tbsp. parsley flakes
2 tbsp. basil
½ tsp. red pepper
black pepper
8 cups chicken bouillon or vegetable stock

Combine all ingredients in a large pot, bring to a boil, cover and simmer for 2–3 hours. Makes 8 (1 cup) servings.

Yogurt Borscht—55 calories

2½ cups beets, shredded
4½ cups vegetable bouillon
6 tbsp. lemon juice
black pepper
low-fat yogurt, plain

Combine beets, beet juice, and bouillon in large pot and bring to a boil. Simmer for 10 minutes, add lemon juice and pepper to taste. Serve hot or chilled, topped with a dollop of yogurt. Makes 6 (1 cup) servings.

Fresh Onion Soup—20 calories

3 med. onions, sliced thin
5 beef bouillon cubes
4 cups water, boiling
¼ tsp. Worcestershire sauce
Parmesan cheese, grated

Add onions, bouillon cubes, and Worcestershire sauce to boiling water, cover, and simmer for 30 minutes. Serve with a sprinkling of grated cheese on top. Makes 9 (1 cup) servings.

Fresh Mushroom Soup—75 calories

2 tbsp. margarine
½ lb. mushrooms, sliced
1 sm. onion, sliced
1 quart chicken broth
1 cup low-fat milk
salt and pepper

Melt margarine in saucepan over medium heat, stir in mushrooms and onions, add liquids and cook over low heat. Season lightly to taste. Makes 6 (1 cup) servings.

Broccoli-Cauliflower Soup—70 calories

1 10-oz. pkg. frozen chopped broccoli
1 10-oz. pkg. frozen cauliflower
1/3 cup onion, chopped
2 chicken bouillon cubes
1½ cups water

3 cups low-fat milk
1 tbsp. cornstarch
pepper, black
¼ cup low-fat cheese, shredded

Cook frozen vegetables with onion and bouillon in the water in a large saucepan for 5 to 8 minutes, or until tender. Do not drain, but puree in blender (only half the mixture at a time). Combine ½ cup of the milk with the cornstarch, add pureed vegetables, and stir in the rest of the milk. Add pepper to taste. Cook in the saucepan, stirring constantly, until thick and bubbly. Continue to cook for 1 to 2 more minutes before adding cheese. Stir until cheese melts. Makes 8 servings.

Pea-Plus Soup—250 calories

1 cup shelled peas
3–4 spinach leaves
5 lettuce leaves
¼ cups leeks, chopped
1 chicken bouillon cube
pepper, black
5/8 cup water
3/8 cup low-fat milk

In large saucepan, combine all ingredients except milk and bring to a boil. Reduce heat, cover, and simmer for 20 minutes. Pour into blender and process until smooth. Sieve into saucepan, add milk, and heat slowly. Serves 3.

Cream of Leftover-Vegetables Soup—65 calories

¼ med. onion, minced
1 celery stalk
½ green onion, minced
¼ cup chicken or vegetable stock
¼ leftover baked potato or ¼ cup mashed potato
½ cup leftover cooked vegetables (broccoli, carrots, tomatoes, peas, green
   beans, corn, cauliflower, zucchini, whatever)
½ cup low-fat milk
1 tbsp. dried skim milk powder
parsley, black pepper

In a small saucepan, sauté onions and celery until transparent in a little of the stock. Add rest of stock, potato, and leftover vegetables, bring to a boil, and simmer for 2 minutes. Remove vegetables with slotted spoon, puree in blender, return to pan. Stir in milk and simmer for 5 minutes, season to taste. Serves 2.

Fresh Berry Soup—115 calories

1 pint fresh strawberries (and/or raspberries, blueberries, others in season)
2 tsp. cornstarch
½ cup orange juice
½ cup red wine
2 tbsp. apple juice concentrate
½ cup low-fat yogurt

Cut berries if large and purée. In a saucepan, blend cornstarch with half of the orange juice, add remaining juice, wine, apple juice and purée. Over medium heat, heat just to boiling, stirring frequently. Remove from heat, cool, and stir in yogurt with a wire whisk. Cover and refrigerate for 2 to 4 hours before serving. Serves 2.

Sandwiches to Savor—Easy as 1-2-3

Sandwiches need not be limited to luncheon meats, tuna, or peanut butter. Using a bit of imagination and a sense of adventure, numerous nutritious ingredients can be combined between bread slices . . . and the types of bread chosen should be quite varied as well. Select from the following lists to create a wide variety of deliciously different sandwiches.

Breads

white	hard roll
wheat	matzoh
cracked wheat	egg bread
oatmeal	cheese bread
raisin	garlic bread
bran	croissant
rye	English muffin
sourdough	hot dog bun
brown bread	hamburger bun
pita	French bread
pumpernickel	Italian bread
whole wheat pita	tortilla
bulkie roll	corn bread
submarine roll	bagel
onion roll	quick breads

Vegetables

lettuce	water chestnuts
tomato	carrots, shredded
onion	cole slaw
green pepper	radishes
zucchini	chicory
mushrooms	endive
spinach	escarole
cucumber	watercress
cabbage, shredded	sauerkraut
sprouts	

Other Fillers

cooked beans	eggs
peanut butter	cooked potato
banana	avocado
raisins	applesauce
cheeses, low-fat	grapes, sliced
cottage cheese, low-fat	chopped liver
fish or seafood	nuts, chopped or sliced (unsalted)
poultry	seeds, unsalted
lean meat	apple, sliced

Extras

chives
jam
jelly
preserves
relish
pickles
hot peppers
mustard
mayonnaise

hot chili sauce
catsup
bean dip
herbs and seasoning
salad dressings, low-fat
margarine
yogurt, low-fat
spicy mustard

Salad Daze—Easy as 1-2-3, too

Just as in sandwich design, tossing a salad can be fast and fun, with delicious, nutritious results. Use a little creativity to prepare unusual and appetizing salads which contain a wide variety of ingredients and the many nutrients which accompany them. Choose from the following lists to spruce up the basic lettuce and tomato salad:

Basics

onion
lettuce
tomato
cucumber
pepper, green
pepper, red

carrots
celery
greens
chicory
endive
escarole

Vegetables

bean sprouts
beets
beans, green or yellow
spinach
mushrooms
cabbage
pickled vegetables
sauerkraut
avocado
asparagus

broccoli
cauliflower
Brussels sprouts
eggplant
zucchini
radishes
watercress
peas
parsley

Additional Ingredients

pineapple chunks
apple, sliced
grapes, sliced
orange, sectioned
Mandarin orange sections
3-bean salad
cole slaw
tofu
garbanzo beans
chick peas
kidney beans

egg, hard boiled
cheese, low-fat
lean meat
poultry
fish and seafood
potato, cooked
garlic clove, crushed
cottage cheese, low-fat
banana, sliced
dried apricots, peaches, pears
peach or pear, sliced

Top It Off

seeds, unsalted
unsalted nuts
alfalfa sprouts
wheat germ
Parmesan cheese grated
raisins
croutons
hot chili peppers
yogurt, low-fat

corn/tortilla chips, crumbled
mint leaves
horseradish
various vinegar
lemon
black pepper
red pepper
salad dressings, low-fat

E-Z Entrées—Keep It Lean

- Meats can be good sources of high quality protein, iron, other minerals and vitamins. However, there is no need to ingest over-sized cuts, nor to opt for those high-fat marbled choices. Eat small portions, stretch meat by serving as an extender with vegetables and/or grains in casseroles, soups, and stews, and be sure to select lean cuts, then trim off all visible fat.
- Prepare meats by baking, boiling, broiling, or roasting using racks to allow fat to drain. Remove skin from poultry, skim fat from soups and stews, and avoid fried meat, poultry, or fish.
- The less expensive cuts are often better buys nutritionally as well. Fish and seafood are low in fat-calories, but high in protein and other nutrients.
- No need to eliminate red meats, but opt more often for the lower fat choices, such as poultry, fish, seafood or meatless meals based around legumes, eggs, low-fat cheeses with vegetables and grains.

Recipes

Pasta with Vegetables—200 calories

2 oz. linguini
1 tbsp. margarine
½ cup broccoli, thin slices
1 sm. carrot, thin slices
¼ cup onion, thin slices
black pepper
garlic powder
3/4 cup mushrooms, sliced
½ 6-oz. pkg. frozen peapods
2 tbsp. dry white wine
Parmesan cheese

Cook linguini in boiling water until tender; drain and keep warm. Melt margarine in small skillet, stir in broccoli, carrot, onion and seasonings, and cook for several minutes until vegetables are tender-crisp. Add mushrooms and cook for 2 more minutes. Add peapods and wine, cover and cook for two minutes. Stir in linguini, toss, and sprinkle with grated cheese. Serves 2.

Lentil and Rice Casserole—200 calories

1½ cups chicken broth
3/8 cup dry lentils
3/8 cup onion, chopped
¼ cup brown rice, uncooked
2 tbsp. dry white wine
oregano, thyme, garlic powder, black pepper
2 oz. low-fat mozzarella cheese, shredded

Combine all ingredients with half of the shredded cheese and bake covered in a small casserole dish at 350 degrees for 1–1½ hours, stirring twice. When lentils and rice are done, uncover and sprinkle with remaining cheese. Bake for 2 to 3 minutes or until cheese is melted. Serves 3.

Vegetable De-Lights—Nutrient Saving Tips

- Buy produce which is fresh, and free from bruising; handle carefully. Wash thoroughly before storing in refrigerator. Wrap in plastic and keep in vegetable bin. Air, heat, and light can destroy some vitamins.
- Avoid soaking vegetables in water, and cook quickly until tender-crisp in small amounts of water or by steaming. Save broth from cooked and canned vegetables for making vegetable stocks. Vitamins and minerals will be lost if the cooking water is thrown out.
- Avoid peeling and paring produce if possible; much of the vitamin value lies in and just underneath the skins.
- Vegetables and fruits with skins and seeds are notable sources of fiber, as well as vitamins and minerals.
- Try stir-frying vegetables in a Chinese wok or in a skillet. By using small amounts of oil, low-calorie and high-nutrient vegetable dishes can be rapidly prepared.
- Use iron skillets to prepare acidic vegetables, such as tomatoes, so that the iron will leach into the food (to add the nutrient iron to your body stores).
- Canned vegetables may be high in sodium, but more and more companies are producing low-sodium alternatives: Read the labels before you buy.
- Frozen vegetables are often better choices than their fresh counterparts because they are packaged at the peak of freshness and less apt to have lost nutrients during storage.

Recipes

Brussels Sprouts 'n' Onions—80 calories

1/3 quart fresh Brussels sprouts
2 tsp. margarine

1 sm. onion, thinly sliced
1 bouillon cube dissolved in ½ cup boiling water
1 tbsp. parsley flakes
pepper, black

Add sprouts to 1 cup boiling water and cook covered for 5 minutes, drain. Heat margarine, onion, stock and pepper in a saucepan and simmer for 5 minutes. Add sprouts, toss, and sprinkle with parsley. Serves 2.

Vegetable Broiler—80 calories

2 tbsp. lemon juice
2 tsp. vegetable oil
1 sm. eggplant, chunks
½ green pepper, chunks
1 tomato, chunks
1 sm. onion, thick slices
6 lg. mushrooms, thick slices

In a large bowl, combine the lemon juice and oil. Add vegetables and marinate, turning often, for an hour or more. Drain, arrange in shallow pan, and broil for 5 minutes. Serves 2.

Baked Beets—25 calories

2–3 lg. beets, ends cut
lemon juice
chives

Wrap beets in foil and bake at 375 degrees for 1 to 1½ hours, or until tender and skin easily slips off. Cut into strips, toss with lemon and chives, serve warm or chilled. Serves 2.

Baked Asparagus—30 calories

½ lb. asparagus, ends cut
lemon juice
chives

Wrap asparagus in foil and bake at 350 degrees for 30 minutes. Sprinkle with lemon juice and chives. Serves 2.

Marinated Mixed Vegetables—50 calories

1 cup carrots, diced
1 cup zucchini, diced
1 cup cauliflower, diced
1 cup broccoli, diced
¼ cup green pepper, diced
2 radishes, sliced
12 cherry tomatoes

Marinade: ¼ cup dry white wine, 1 cup plain low-fat yogurt, 1 garlic clove (minced), oregano and black pepper to taste.

In a large bowl, combine vegetables. Pour on marinade mixture, stirring until vegetables are well coated. Cover and refrigerate for at least 2 hours. Makes 8 (½ cup) servings.

Orange-Cucumber Salad Mix—55 calories

½ cup cucumber, thin slices
1 orange, peeled and sectioned
¼ cup green pepper, chopped
black pepper, parsley flakes
¼ cup low-fat yogurt
thyme

In a small mixing bowl, toss cucumber, orange and green pepper with black pepper and parsley to taste. Combine yogurt with thyme and spoon onto salad. Toss lightly, cover and chill. Serve on salad greens or lettuce bed. Serves 2.

Baked Sweets—80 calories

½ med. sweet potato
nutmeg
cinnamon

Scrub potato thoroughly and bake at 350 degrees for 30 to 40 minutes, or until soft. Remove from oven, cut an "X" to let out steam, sprinkle with spices. May serve with a dollop of low-fat yogurt, if desired.

Braised Red Cabbage—120 calories

1/3 cup chicken stock
½ cup onions, chopped
1 med. red cabbage, shredded
5 sweet apples, peeled and sliced
½ cup cider vinegar
½ cup chicken stock
½ cup red wine
1/3 cup apple juice concentrate
nutmeg, allspice

Heat the 1/3 cup of stock in a casserole dish. Add onions and cook over medium heat for 5 minutes. Add cabbage, apples, vinegar, and the ½ cup of stock. Simmer for 2 hours, then add rest of ingredients, and cook for 30 more minutes. Makes 7 (1 cup) servings.

Dessert Do's—Sweet Talk

Since you know from reading the previous chapters that food is meant to provide pleasure as well as nutrients, there is no reason for you to feel guilty about enjoying dessert. A slice of birthday cake, a piece of pumpkin pie, a candy cane, or Valentine's Day chocolates are all part of our social customs. As long as your diet does not consist entirely of tea and cookies, there certainly is nothing wrong with including favorite foods in your diet plan. Some of the more nutritious sweets include the following choices:

Peanut butter cookies
Oatmeal-raisin cookies
Fig bars
Date bars
Molasses cookies
Carrot cake (without icing)
Sesame candies

Apple crisp, Betty, cobbler
Brandied and baked fruits
Fruited gelatin
Puddings (especially made with
    low-fat milk)
Ice cream (plain, fruit, with nuts)
Ice milk and frozen yogurt

Recipes

Pineapple Boats—90 calories

1 med. ripe pineapple
4 lg. fresh strawberries
4 tsp. liqueur

Slice pineapple in half lengthwise, then cut into quarters. With a flexible knife, slice fruit away from shell and cut crosswise into bite size wedges. Arrange in pineapple shell and pour on liqueur. Wrap in foil and chill. Serve with strawberry garnish. Makes 4 servings.

Charcoal Grilled Apples—around 90 calories

Core an apple and place in center of aluminum foil. Stuff center with raisins, seal up, and place on grill over hot coals. Cook for 10 to 15 minutes.

Fruited Gelatin—35 calories

1 cup water
1 cup orange juice
1 envelope unflavored gelatin
1 cup pineapple tidbits

Combine water and juice with gelatin in saucepan. Stir over low heat until gelatin dissolves. Cool and pour into mold; add pineapple. Chill until firm. Makes 6 servings.

Apple Crisp—170 calories

1 cup rolled oats
1 cup whole wheat flour
½ cup Grape-Nuts
2 tsp. cinnamon
2 cups apple juice
2 cups apples, sliced
½ cup raisins
1 tbsp. lemon juice
2 tsp. cornstarch

For crust, combine oats, flour, cereal and 1 tsp. cinnamon. Stir in 1 cup juice until mixture holds together. Press half of mixture into greased 9-inch square pan to line bottom and sides. Bake at 350 degrees for 5 minutes. For fillings, combine apples, raisins, lemon juice, and cornstarch with 1 cup juice and 1 tsp. cinnamon. Bring to a boil and simmer for 10 minutes. Remove apples and raisins with slotted spoon and place on crust. Continue cooking juice at higher heat until sauce thickens. Pour over fruit, crumble remaining crust on top, and bake at 375 degrees for 30 minutes. Makes 9 servings.

Whipped Berry Gelatin—8 calories

1 4-serving envelope of low-calorie strawberry or raspberry-flavored gelatin
1 cup boiling water
1 cup low-calorie lemon/lime-flavored soft drink

Dissolve the gelatin in boiling water, cool to room temperature, stir in soft drink and chill until partially set. Beat in a mixing bowl until light and fluffy, spoon into serving dishes and chill until firm. Makes 4 servings.

Lemon Ice—105 calories

½ cup sugar
½ cup boiling water
1 cup cold water
¼ tsp. lemon peel, shredded
½ cup lemon juice

Dissolve sugar in boiling water, add cold water and lemon, and pour into ice cube trays. Freeze for 2 hours or until almost firm. Break into pieces in mixing bowl and beat until fluffy. Freeze again until almost firm, and serve in 4 small bowls.

Lemon Cupcakes—65 calories

2 eggs, separated
½ tsp. salt
½ cup sugar
1 tsp. lemon juice
½ cup flour

Beat egg whites with salt until stiff. Gradually add sugar, beating after each addition. In a separate bowl, beat yolks with lemon juice until thickened and fold into stiffened white. Carefully fold in flour until well blended and spoon into lined muffin tins, filling 7/8 full. Bake at 400 degrees for 10–12 minutes. Makes 12 cupcakes.

Thirst Quenchers—Light on Liquids

Although you may not realize it, the beverages you drink may be serving as a significant source of hidden calories. You need an average intake of 1 or 2 quarts of fluid per day, but if your choice of drink is calorie-laden, then you may be gulping down more than you think. Some tips are listed below for keeping the caloric contribution of your liquid intake on the lighter side:

- Nothing beats a cold glass of water (0 calories).
- Club soda, mineral water, and sparkling waters cost more than tap water, but are non-caloric as well.
- Diet soft drinks come in all sorts of flavors and varieties, with different types of non-nutritive sweeteners, and with or without caffeine.
- Tomato juice is lower in calories than fruit juices, and low-sodium varieties are available.
- Opt for dry wine or "light" beers over the high calorie "booze" alternatives; if you drink mixed drinks, remember that the mixers, as well as the liquors, provide calories.
- Low-fat or skim milk are relatively easy to develop a taste for, and are rich in nutritional value.
- Cream, non-dairy creamers, and sugar can add quite a few calories to your coffee or tea; opt for black, or switch to low-fat milk and non-nutritive sweeteners.

Recipes

Vegetable Refresher—50 calories

¼ med. cucumber, peeled and seeded
1 cup vegetable juice cocktail, cold
½ cup buttermilk

Cut cucumber into small pieces and combine with liquids in blender. Cover and blend until cucumber is pureed. Makes 2 large servings.

Sangria—75 calories

1 orange, halved
1 lemon, halved
1 750-ml. bottle rosé wine
2 tbsp. honey
1 apple, cut into wedges
2 cups carbonated water, cold

Chill half the orange and half the lemon for garnish; squeeze juice from other halves and mix with wine and honey before chilling. Slice chilled orange and lemon into wheels, add apples to wine mixture. Before serving, mix with carbonated water. Makes about 12 (4 oz.) servings.

Pineapple-Lemon Smoothie—175 calories

½ cup crushed pineapple (in juice)
½ cup lemon yogurt, low-fat
¼ cup low-fat milk
2–3 ice cubes

Blend crushed pineapple with juice, yogurt and milk until smooth. Add ice cubes, one at a time, blending after each until icy. Serve in tall glass, chilled.

Fruit Cooler—95 calories

1 med. orange
1/3 sm. banana, sliced
3 tbsp. white grape juice
1 tsp. lemon juice

Squeeze juice from orange and combine with remaining ingredients. Blend and serve.

Cranberry Warmup—80 calories

½ cup low-calorie cranberry juice cocktail
¼ cup pineapple juice
allspice, cloves, nutmeg
cinnamon stick

Combine all ingredients in small saucepan and slowly bring to a boil. Reduce heat, cover, and simmer for 20 minutes. Strain out spices and serve in a mug.

Peach-Yogurt with a Kick—75 calories

1 cup low-fat yogurt, plain
¼ cup peach brandy

1 10-oz. pkg. frozen peaches, partly thawed
nutmeg

Combine yogurt with brandy, add peaches and blend until smooth. Pour into 5 tall glasses and sprinkle with nutmeg before serving.

Phyllis Diller and George Burns: Health Through Humor

One way to remain eternally young is to enjoy a daily dose of laughter. Phyllis Diller and George Burns are two very visible examples of extended youth through humor. Plastic surgery, as Ms. Diller does not hesitate to admit, can also do wonders!

Phyllis Diller is currently following a very restrictive diet regimen prescribed for her by a nutrition "doctor." Some of the dietary rules advocated by her strict new diet plan include:

- No sugar
- No tea, coffee, soft drinks, cocoa
- No fried foods
- No prepared meats
- No alcohol
- No preservatives or additives
- No food to be eaten more often than every 4 days (i.e., oranges on Monday cannot be eaten again until Friday)
- Mineral water only

Fortunately, Ms. Diller is able to retain a sense of humor and zest for living in spite of her dull diet. In fact, she admits to "cheating a little with alcohol"—who can blame her?

George Burns, on the other hand, advocates a "flexible" diet as illustrated below. Burns emphasizes the importance of exercise, especially walking. Although Phyllis Diller finds exercise "boring," George Burns says, "Walking is even easier than making a martini . . . you don't even need an olive."*

The George Burns Seven-Day Diet*

Breakfast: 4 prunes with low-fat milk
2 cups coffee, black

There are other fruits I could eat for breakfast, but I prefer prunes because they've got more wrinkles than I have. I tried raisins once and they have good wrinkles, too. In fact, they have excellent wrinkles. But four raisins isn't much for breakfast, even for me. I wish they'd start making bananas with wrinkles; I'd like to try one of them.

Lunch: Bowl of soup
1 slice French bread, toasted
1 cup coffee, black

This is very flexible. If you haven't got French bread, rye bread is fine, or white bread, or rolls, or fruitcake. And it doesn't have to be a bowl of soup and a cup of coffee. It can be a bowl of coffee and a cup of soup. Whatever makes you happy. As I said, this is a very flexible diet.

Dinner: Bowl of soup	Green peas
Mixed green salad	1 slice bread, buttered
Roast chicken	1 cup coffee, black
Rice	Cookies

This is my big meal of the day. If I'm still hungry, I might include the one prune left over from breakfast. And the cookies must be very crisp so they make a noise in my mouth when I eat them. It sounds like applause, so I can eat and take bows at the same time.

Despite their different ideas on diet and exercise, both of these popular comedians have incorporated one of the keys to longevity into their own individual lifestyles: love of life. As George Burns cleverly explains, "Dying is not popular; it's never caught on. That's understandable—it upsets your daily routine and leaves you with too much time on your hands."* Laughter may be the best *preventive* medicine after all!

*From Burns' *How to Live to Be 100—Or More* (GP Putnam's Sons, 1983).

LIVING LONGER AND ENJOYING IT MORE

According to Harvard's well-known behavioral scientist, B.F. Skinner, old age need not be a "badly written last act" in the live play of your life. Instead, by setting up a stage of life which is supportive of good emotional and physical health, "You will undoubtedly be admired—not only for a great performance, but for writing a last act that plays so well."

Dr. Skinner—who is over 80 years old—recently published a book on growing old with dignity and self-esteem entitled *Enjoy Old Age* (W.W. Norton, 1983). With co-author, Dr. Margaret E. Vaughan, a consultant on aging, Dr. Skinner outlines a number of methods for composing the last scene of your life as a true masterpiece, one filled with the joys of living. In reference to nutrition, the authors suggest the establishment of regular meals and a daily exercise plan. Sound familiar?

Another book on growing old well was written by a professor at the University of Pennsylvania, Dr. Joseph G. Richardson: *Long Life and How to Reach It* includes information on the avoidable causes of disease, environmental factors in health and illness, exercise, sleep, and old age. Dr. Richardson does not present readers with full directions for preserving good health, but does give "some general rules for the protection of our valuable bodies."

Diet and nutrition are mentioned often throughout the book, and two chapters are entirely devoted to desirable dietary practices: "Food and How to Digest It" emphasizes the importance of obtaining a varied diet which includes moderate amounts of different foods. Another chapter on "Impurities in Food and Drink, and How to Detect Them" discusses food safety.

The following list of selected quotes from these two chapters illustrates the general theme of Dr. Richardson's health advice:

1. Year after year, from the cradle to the grave, we all go on violating the plainest and simplest laws of health, at the temptation of cooks, caterers, and confectioners, whose share in shortening the average term of human life is probably nearly equal to that of the combined armies and navies of the world.
2. In average health, the amount of food taken into the stomach might safely be left to the control of the appetite, were it not for the machinations of cooks, who contrive to delude and entrap our natural guide in this vitally important affair into all sorts of immoderate excesses.
3. Of course, we ought all to strive to overcome constipation by laxative articles of diet, such as bran bread, fruit-fresh or dried—and by suitable exercise.
4. Degeneration of arteries, etc., is a common and serious mode of decay in advanced life, due in part, perhaps, to errors in diet.
5. Another important change very liable to accompany advancing years is the excessive deposit of fat which, unfortunately, often occurs just at the time when the muscular powers are deteriorating a little, and the corpulent condition, therefore, interferes with taking sufficient bodily exercise to ensure uninterrupted good health. This tendency may be diminished by attention to diet.

These statements appear to be accurate descriptions of the current American tendency for dietary overindulgence coupled with the general lack of physical activity. Yet *Long Life and How To Reach It* was written over a century ago and was published in 1880! Thus, the self-indulgent lifestyle which is typical of most Americans in today's society is not at all new, nor does it represent a serious degeneration from the "good old days."

We are a nation which has long been susceptible to the temptations of rich foods, alcoholic beverages, and lazy living. Yet we constantly seek to live longer, healthier lives—perhaps because we want to continue to indulge ourselves for as long as possible. Even though Dr. Richardson's advice is over 100 years old, much of it is as applicable today as it was during his time.

According to Drs. Skinner and Richardson, as well as today's gerontologists and health professionals, it is possible to live to be fifty or sixty years *young*. . . or seventy, eighty, ninety or more. One can also be forty years *old*, or even thirty years *old*. The choice is—and always has been—ours to make. (NOTE: *Life span* is the uppermost limit gauged as possible for human life to last, while *life expectancy* is the reality of our cultural and environmental influences—for males, this now exceeds 71 years and for females, 78.) The oldest human on record was a Japanese male who lived to be 114. Claims of achieving greater ages have never been proven, and are usually highly exaggerated, mainly for media attention.

In this regard, "Life Extension" formulas—and the book under that title—play on our desires for long life and, with exaggerated claims, have drawn much media regard. The best-seller *Life Extension* is based on self-experimentation using 33 different supplements (minerals, vitamins, amino acids, food additives, even prescription drugs) plus "antacids as needed"—which may be often. The cost of following such a regimen was estimated in the "Harvard Medical School of Health Letter" to be $64 a day. This means that each of the "extra" years (from age 80 to 140) would cost one $39,000 in supplements; and if one purchased enough of these supplements for a century of life, it would cost over $2 million!

The jacket photo of the two authors of *Life Extension*, an 858-page tome, is designed so that prospective buyers will believe that the young, long-haired, unconventional-looking duo have combined laboratory and ultramodern technology skills (Durk Pearson is holding a beaker in an arm swathed in Indian jewelry, Sandy Shaw is holding a computer printout, and the screen on their home computer module is aglow with figures) to come up with THE WAY to "enjoy the pleasure and stamina, the vitality and strength, of youth—longer." A mere $22.50 does not seem like an outrageous fee "for anyone . . . who seeks greater youthfulness" to shell out for advice on the accomplishment of the following elusive feats:

> slowing your own aging while improving your current health, mental abilities, sexual function and pleasure;
> getting most of the benefits of exercise in a few minutes per day;
> and reducing your risks from smoking and drinking, even if you don't quit.

Each of the authors (who prefer to be called by their first names) has an undergraduate degree in science, but discontinued formal education in favor of self-experimentation and self-directed research. Durk and Sandy are not at all shy about allowing the public to examine their personal lives, including dietary habits, "exercise" techniques (with several centerfolds of the two, scantily clad, posed in body-building stances), and sex life. But in "sharing" their own anti-aging program with readers, Durk and Sandy are foresighted enough to caution us with dozens of disclaimers, including:

> The use of prescription drugs and large doses of nutrients for the improvement of health in normal people is still experimental. Some applications of scientific findings we report are based on results in a small number of people. Be sure to have regular clinical laboratory tests if you plan to experiment with any of these substances yourself;

None of the nutrients and prescription drugs we use is FDA-approved as a therapy for life extension; and

Do not imagine that any of our suggestions can substitute for your doctor's treatment of serious disorders . . . do not stop your prescribed medications, and make sure you consult your doctor about adding our suggestions!

Some of the "health" advice contained in Durk and Sandy's book would be humorous if it were not so dangerous. The so-called "Life Extension nutrients" are not all nutrients and some are actually drugs:

a prescription drug containing canthaxanthin—which is available in Canada but unapproved by the U.S. FDA—as a skin-coloring agent for those who want a suntan without ever seeing the sun;
the prescription drug Hydergine (prescribed for serious mental disabilities) for removal of "liver spots" and a generally slowed aging process;
L-Dopa (prescribed for Parkinson's disease) for increased life span, energy, and "motivation" to exercise;
Hydergine (in tablet form taken sublingually) to protect against smoker's cough;
Dilantin as chewable children's tablets (prescribed for seizures) during cigarette smoking "withdrawal";
Vasopressin nasal spray to improve intelligence; and
topical sex hormones to enhance sex drive.

The non-prescription non-nutritive medication/supplements advised for a variety of ills include: RNA, lecithin, choline, bioflavonoids, and BHA and BHT (approved as food additives, not dietary supplements). Arthritis sufferers are advised to get a waterbed, the heartbroken are informed about the "curative" effects of chocolate, and the overweight are told they need only exercise for two minutes a week.

The actual nutrients Durk and Sandy recommend have to be considered as drugs when taken as self-prescribed supplements and in excessive doses. Durk and Sandy's personal formula includes megadoses of vitamins A, C, and several B's (plus calcium pantothenate, which they incorrectly label as "vitamin B_5"), as well as zinc, selenium and certain amino acids. In combination with their prescription drugs and non-nutritive supplements, Durk and Sandy ingest the costly daily total of 33 items, plus a diet rich in eggs, whole milk, beef, butter, and sweets, as well as the "antacids as desired." Potential readers of this ridiculous book would be wiser to take only the antacids, or save their money to spend on enjoyable items—travel, activity, food and fun—during their long, healthy, unsupplemented lifetimes.

Why contribute *your* hard-earned money to the estimated $2 billion wasted annually on anti-aging "remedies," currently the fastest growing area of the booming business in medical quackery?

Like a good wine which improves with age, so can you. All you need is a healthful lifestyle coupled with a youthful attitude. Why not transform your "last act" into a delightful comedy of life with the enjoyment of living which can be shared with others, with people who will toast you always as a vintage model with an engine that just wouldn't stop!

Two Decades of White House Diets

Over age 50 himself, Executive Chef Henry Haller exudes excitement and enthusiasm when he recounts the myriad menus and different dining habits of the first families he has served. Summoned to the White House in 1966 by Lady Bird Johnson, the Swiss-born chef left his executive position at the splendid Sheraton Hotel Complex in New York City to begin a lengthy stint in a totally unique environ. Nearly twenty years have passed, but Chef Haller is still able to describe in fascinating detail the gala state dinners of the Johnson presidential term, and can convey with equal eagerness the eating habits of the current presidency.

In examining the eating styles of the past five presidents, their families and guests, a distinct trend emerges: The White House menus have gradually evolved from elaborate repasts of numerous courses into simpler meals of far lighter fare. The emphasis on healthful (yet enjoyable!) eating has become quite distinct at this time, whereas earlier menus featured fancy foodstuffs of impressive quantity and rich, expensive quality. Today's typical White House dinner is attractive to behold, yet sensibly affordable and nutritious. One can only imagine that the menu choices of five of the most influential men in America's history can serve as illuminating reflections of both the state of nutrition consciousness in this country during these eras, and the attitudes of these important individuals toward food and health. Let's take a look at some sample menus which typify the meals that adorn(ed) the White House dinner table:

Lyndon B. Johnson (1964–1968)

Breakfast	*Lunch*	*Dinner*
fresh fruit juice or melons in season	hearty beef barley soup	roast rib of beef
chipped beef on toast	crackers	Yorkshire pudding
coffee	tapioca pudding with fresh fruit slices	mustard greens
		tossed salad
		Spanish crème

President Johnson had a hearty appetite and constantly struggled to be a more controlled, disciplined eater. He was not shy about helping himself to seconds during meals, including the state dinners at which extravagant, lengthy menus—appetizers, several courses, salad and dessert—were customary. The Johnsons actually preferred plain food without fancy decorations, and occasionally enjoyed down-home Texas-style meals such as chili and corn bread. President Johnson was especially enthusiastic about the rather rich desserts prepared daily for his well-stocked dinner table, but he always insisted on having very fresh, very ripe fruit as well.

Richard M. Nixon (1968–1974)

Breakfast	*Lunch*	*Dinner*
grapefruit half ready-to-eat cereal with skim milk coffee	cottage cheese with fresh fruit or seafood salad plate iced tea	scaloppini of veal in marsala sauce rice pilaf steamed broccoli spears cold lemon soufflé

The Nixons preferred simple food served at regular times without the traditional course after course after course. Thus, the typical menus during Nixon's term eliminated fancy foodstuffs, appetizers, and most desserts in favor of rather plain fare. The Nixons forfeited eating excitement in favor of careful waist watching.

Gerald R. Ford (1974–1976)

Breakfast	*Lunch*	*Dinner*
English muffins, toasted (on Sundays:) waffles with sour cream and strawberries coffee	hot consommé cold salmon paté homemade rolls fresh fruit	sliced double sirloin steak baked stuffed potatoes steamed red cabbage watercress salad apple tart

The Fords also like simple food, but President Ford ate quite heartily. In fact, although the menus centered around a small range of his basic favorites (including homebaked bread, sliced and toasted), President Ford would eat almost anything on the menu—from stuffed peppers or cabbage to lasagna or casserole. Daily swims helped to keep him trim in spite of his ardent appetite.

James E. Carter (1976–1980)

Breakfast	*Lunch*	*Dinner*
orange juice (at 6:00 am) ready-to-eat cereal with skim milk coffee	vegetable soup toasted cheese sandwich skim milk fruit	(Wednesdays) Southern fried chicken corn bread steamed ochra tossed greens fresh berries in season

The Carters were always very careful about reducing waste— energy, finances, and food—as they strongly believed in and practiced modest living. A disciplined family, President and Mrs. Carter both jogged daily and they preferred a narrow repertoire of Southern foodstuffs served at regular hours without any fancy fanfare. Yet, they were always open to trying new menu items, allowing the kitchen staff to expand the menus with creativity and imagination. One of Mrs. Carter's favorite recipes was not to Chef Haller's liking, but many guests seemed to enjoy this unusual appetizer and often asked him for the recipe: Mrs. Carter's "cheese ring" consisted of a circular mold made from cheddar cheese, onions, mayonnaise and pecans, the center filled with strawberry jam(!?!).

Ronald Reagan (1980–1984 and 1984–present)

Breakfast	*Lunch*	*Dinner*
mixed fruit cup grapefruit juice cereal or egg (poached, soft-boiled, scrambled) whole wheat toast decaffeinated coffee	seafood salad plate herbed pita bread baked fresh pear iced tea	baked breast of chicken with fresh black cherries wild rice with walnuts steamed green asparagus spears pineapple sorbet

The Reagans are also a disciplined couple, but they enjoy experimenting with new and interesting foodstuffs. Mrs. Reagan is very interested in food and cooking, but she is careful to control their nutritional and caloric intakes. Attractive, colorful meals which are prepared lightly and presented gracefully are the norm in today's White House dining room.

Of all the Administrations with whom he has worked, Chef Haller has found that the Reagans show the most interest in the food they eat and the most concern for the nutritional value of the meals which are served. Haller has prepared daily meals during five different terms with five individual dietary patterns: geographical, familial, religious and cultural influences have all contributed to the menu construct for each of these President's dinner table, while personal likes and dislikes, attitudes and behaviors have also helped to dictate the menu design. If one considers the White House to be representative of the nation's households, the dietary trend in America appears to have veered away from expensive and expansive feasts toward simpler, more nutritious, yet very palatable fare. From the White House to our own dining rooms, it appears that more and more Americans are eating sensibly, healthfully, and enjoyably.

Appendix A:

RDA's

Recommended Dietary Allowances for Older Adults*

	Age (years)	Weight (kg)	Weight (lb)	Height (cm)	Height (in)	Protein (g)	Fat-Soluble Vitamins Vita-min A (µg RE)	Vita-min D (µg)	Vita-min E (mg α-TE)	Water-Soluble Vitamins Vita-min C (mg)	Thia-min (mg)	Ribo-flavin (mg)	Niacin (mg NE)	Vita-min B-6 (mg)	Fola-cin (µg)	Vitamin B-12 (µg)	Minerals Cal-cium (mg)	Phos-phorus (mg)	Mag-nesium (mg)	Iron (mg)	Zinc (mg)	Iodine (µg)
Males	11–14	45	99	157	62	45	1000	10	8	50	1.4	1.6	18	1.8	400	3.0	1200	1200	350	18	15	150
	15–18	66	145	176	69	56	1000	10	10	60	1.4	1.7	18	2.0	400	3.0	1200	1200	400	18	15	150
	19–22	70	154	177	70	56	1000	7.5	10	60	1.5	1.7	19	2.2	400	3.0	800	800	350	10	15	150
	23–50	70	154	178	70	56	1000	5	10	60	1.4	1.6	18	2.2	400	3.0	800	800	350	10	15	150
	51 +	70	154	178	70	56	1000	5	10	60	1.2	1.4	16	2.2	400	3.0	800	800	350	10	15	150
Females	11–14	46	101	157	62	46	800	10	8	50	1.1	1.3	15	1.8	400	3.0	1200	1200	300	18	15	150
	15–18	55	120	163	64	46	800	10	8	60	1.1	1.3	14	2.0	400	3.0	1200	1200	300	18	15	150
	19–22	55	120	163	64	44	800	7.5	8	60	1.1	1.3	14	2.0	400	3.0	800	800	300	18	15	150
	23–50	55	120	163	64	44	800	5	8	60	1.0	1.2	13	2.0	400	3.0	800	800	300	18	15	150
	51 +	55	120	163	64	44	800	5	8	60	1.0	1.2	13	2.0	400	3.0	800	800	300	10	15	150

Mean Heights and Weights and Recommended Energy Intake*

Category	Age (years)	Weight (kg)	Weight (lb)	Height (cm)	Height (in.)	Energy Needs (with range) (kcal)	Energy Needs (with range)	(MJ)
Males	23–50	70	154	178	70	2700	(2300–3100)	11.3
	51–75	70	154	178	70	2400	(2000–2800)	10.1
	76+	70	154	178	70	2050	(1650–2450)	8.6
Females	23–50	55	120	163	64	2000	(1600–2400)	8.4
	51–75	55	120	163	64	1800	(1400–2200)	7.6
	76+	55	120	163	64	1600	(1200–2000)	6.7

*Adapted from Recommended Dietary Allowances, Ninth Edition, Washington, DC: National Academy of Sciences, 1980.

Appendix B:
Recommended Reading

Normal Nutrition and Diet for Later Years

Aronson, V. Thirty Days to Better Nutrition, Doubleday, 1984.

Hamilton, E. and Whitney, E. Nutrition—Concepts and Controversies, West Publishing Co., 1982.

Reader's Digest. Eat Better, Live Better, The Reader's Digest Association, Inc., 1982.

Stare, F. and Aronson, V. Dear Dr. Stare: What Should I Eat?, George F. Stickley Co., 1982.

Stare, F. and Aronson, V. Your Basic Guide to Nutrition, George F. Stickley, Co., 1983.

Stare, F. and McWilliams, M. Living Nutrition, 4th Ed., John Wiley & Sons, 1983.

Stare, F. and McWilliams, M. Nutrition for Good Health, 2nd Ed., George F. Stickley Co., 1982.

Alfin-Slater, R. and Kritchevsky, D. Nutrition and the Adult, Plenum Press, 1980.

Winick, M. (ed.). Nutrition and Aging, John Wiley & Sons, 1976.

Watkin, D. Handbook of Nutrition, Health, and Aging, Noyes Publications, 1983.

Natow, A. and Heslin, N. Nutrition for the Prime of Your Life, McGraw-Hill, 1983.

Ontario Dietetic Association. The Nuts and Bolts of Nutrition. Ontario Hospital Association, 1980.

Posner, B. Nutrition and the Elderly, Lexington Books, 1979.

McGill, M. The 50 Plus Good Sense Diet, McLean-Hunter, 1982.

Norris, R. and Powell, J. Easy-to-Chew and Easy-on-Salt, Cornwall Books, 1982.

Hsu, J. and Davis, R. (eds.) Handbook of Geriatric Nutrition: Principles and Applications for Nutrition and Diet in Aging, Noyes Publications, 1981.

Klinger, J. Mealtime Manual for People with Disabilities and the Aging, Campbell Soup Corporation, 1978.

Lewis, C. Nutrition—Nutritional Considerations for the Elderly, F. A. Davis Company, 1978.

American Dietetic Association, Patient Nutritional Care in Long-Term Facilities, 1977.

Weight Control

Katahn, M. The 200-Calorie Solution, W.W. Norton and Co., 1982.

Mirkin, G. Getting Thin, Little, Brown and Co., 1983.

Schwartz, B. Diets Don't Work!, Breakthru Publishing, 1982.

Simonson, M. and Heilman, J. The Complete University Medical Diet, Rawson Assoc., 1983.

Stern, J. and Deneberg, R. The Fast Food Diet, Prentice-Hall, 1980.

Weinsier, R. L., Johnson, M. H. and Doleys, D. M. Time Calorie Displacement, George F. Stickley Company, 1983.

Wood, P. California Diet and Exercise Program, Anderson World Books, Inc. 1983.

Trabella, N. Behavior Modification for Weight Control in the Elderly, Acacia Nutrition Program (104 East Plate, Colorado Springs, CO 80901), 1983.

Nutrition and Exercise

Bayrd, N. and Quilter, C. Food for Champions, Houghton-Mifflin, 1982.
Clark, N. The Athlete's Kitchen, CBI Publishing, 1981.
Darden, E. Nautilus Nutrition Book, Contemporary Books, 1981.
Darden E, Your Guide to Physical Fitness, George F. Stickley Company, 1982.
Katch, F. and McArdle, W. Nutrition, Weight Control, and Exercise, Lea & Febiger, 1983.
Powell, B. Blake Powell's Well-Fit Book, George F. Stickley Company, 1983.
Adult Physical Fitness and the Fitness Challenge in Later Years. (Available from Consumer Information Center, Department G, Pueblo, CO 81009) 1980.
An Introduction to Physical Fitness and Walking for Exercise and Pleasure, (Available from President's Council on Physical Fitness and Sport, Washington, D.C., 20201), 1980.

Food Faddism

Barrett, S. The Health Robbers, 2nd, Ed., George F. Stickley Co., 1980.
Consumer Reports. Health Quackery, Consumers Union, 1980.
Deutsch, R. The New Nuts Among the Berries, Bull Publishing Co., 1977.
Herbert, V. Nutrition Cultism, George F. Stickley Co., 1980.
Herbert, V. and Barrett, S. Vitamins and "Health" Foods, George F. Stickley Co., 1981.
Marshall, C. Vitamins and Minerals: Help or Harm? George F. Stickley Co., 1983.
Tyler, V. The Honest Herbal, George F. Stickley Co., 1982.

Cookbooks

Eshelman, F. and Winston, M. The American Heart Association Cookbook, David McKay Co., 1979.
Middleton, K. and Hess, M. The Art of Cooking for the Diabetic, Contemporary Books, 1976.
Polak, J. Fat and Calorie Controlled Meals, George F. Stickley Company, 1982.
Simmons, R. The Never-Say Diet Cookbook, Warner Books, 1983.
White, A. The Family Health Cookbook, David McKay, Co., 1980.

Cookbooks: Pamphlets

Washbon, M. Cooking for One: In the Senior Years, An Extension Publication of the New York State College of Human Ecology, Cornell University, Ithaca, NY.
Mindman, M. Cooking for Two: In Leisure Years, Clemson University Cooperative Extension Service, Clemson, S. C., (H. E. Circular 243.)
Davis, D. and McGeary, B. Cooking for Two, Program Aid No. 1043, Food and Nutrition Service, U. S. Dept. of Agriculture. (Available from Superintendent of Documents, U. S. Government Printing Office, Washington, D.C. 20402.)
Senior Citizens, Inc. Senior Citizens Cook Alone—And Like It. (Available from Senior Citizens, Inc., 147 East State Street, Ithaca, NY 14850.)

Craig, D. The Single Burner Chef Cookbook, New Hampshire Network (Box 2, Durham, NH 03824).
Eats in My Room, Department of Social and Health Services, Health Services Division, P.O. Box 1788, Olympia, WA 98504.

Selected Topics

Aronson, V. and Fitzgerald, B. Guidebook for Nutrition Counselors, Christopher Publishing House, 1980.
Arthritis Foundation, The Truth About Diet and Arthritis, (The Arthritis Foundation, 3400 Peachtree Road NE, Atlanta, GA 30326), 1982.
Caldwell, L., Nutrition Education for the Patient, George F. Stickley Company, 1984.
Barrett, S. and Rovin, S. The Tooth Robbers, George F. Stickley Co., 1980.
Criswell, C., Group Feeding, George F. Stickley Company, 1983.
Dong, F., All About Food Allergy, George F. Stickley Company, 1984.
Hartbarger, D. C. and Hartbarger, N. J., Eating for the Eighties, George F. Stickley Company, 1981.
Notelovitz, M. and Ware, M. Stand Tall! The Informed Woman's Guide to Preventing Osteoporosis, Triad Publishing Co., 1982.
Sutnick, M., Nutrition and Women's Health, George F. Stickley Company, 1984.
Wilson, N. L. and Wilson, R. H., Please Pass the Salt, George F. Stickley Company, 1983.
Stare, F. and Aronson, V.R. Executive Diet, Christopher Publishing House, 1985.

Selected Topics: Pamphlets

Nutrition Education for the Elderly, Virginia Council on Health and Medical Care, P.O. Box 12363, Central Station, Richmond, VA 23241.
A Guide to Medical Self-Care and Self-Help Groups for the Elderly, U. S. Dept. of Health, Education, and Welfare, NIH Publication No. 80-1687, (Available from the Superintendent of Documents, U. S. Government Printing Office, Washington, D.C. 20402).
Eat and Keep Healthy After 60, Home Economics Service, Community Service Society, 105 East 52nd Street, New York, NY 10010.
Walker, M. and Hill, M. Food Guide for Older Folks, U. S. Dept. of Agriculture, Home and Garden Bulletin No. 17. (Available from the Superintendent of Documents, U. S. Government Printing Office, Washington, D.C. 20402).
Meal Planning for the Golden Years, General Mills, Inc., Nutrition Service, Dept. 5, 9200 Wayzata Blvd., Minneapolis, MN 55440.
Nutrition and the Adult: Suggestions that May Make You Feel Better, available from The New Englander Gerontology Center, 15 Garrison Ave., Durham, NH 03824.
Grodd, F. Your Retirement Food Guide, American Association of Retired Persons and National Retired Teachers Association, 215 Long Beach Blvd., Long Beach, CA 90801.
To Your Health—In Your Second Fifty Years, National Dairy Council, 111 N. Canal Street, Chicago, IL 60606.
Grand Food for Grandparents—Or Those Who Could Be, Tennessee Commission on Aging, Capitol Tower Apartment, 510 Gay Street, Nashville, TN 37219.

Now I Can Eat Nutritious, Low Cost, Convenient Food in My Room, Bureau of Aging, Washington State Department of Social and Health Services, P.O. Box 1788, Olympia, WA 98504.

A Guide for Food and Nutrition in Later Years, Society for Nutrition Education, 1736 Franklin Street, Oakland, CA 94612.

An Older Consumer's Guide to a Healthful Diet on a Low Budget, Blue Cross and Blue Shield Association, Consumer Affairs, 676 St. Clair, Chicago, IL 60611.

Special Report on Aging 1980, US Department of Health and Human Services, NIH Publication No. 80-2135. (Available from the Superintendent of Documents, US Government Printing Office, Washington, DC 20402).

Watkin, D. Aging, Nutrition, and the Continuation of Health Care. Office of State and Community Programs, Administration on Aging, Dept. of Health, Education, and Welfare, Washington, DC 20201.

Warner-Reitz, A. Healthy Lifestyles for Seniors. Meal for Millions/Freedom from Hunger Foundation, 815 Second Avenue, Suite 1001, New York, NY 10017.

For Sources of Nutrition Education Materials

Colleges and Universities—Depts. of Nutrition, Health Sciences, and Home Economics.

Metropolitan Life Insurance Co., Health and Welfare Division, 1 Madison Avenue, New York, NY 10010.

Government Agencies/National Professional Organizations

Food and Drug Administration, 5600 Fisher Lane, Rockville, MD 20852.

Food and Nutrition Information and Education Resources Center, National Agricultural Library, Room 304, Beltsville, MD 20705.

National Institute on Aging, National Institutes of Health, Bethesda, MD 20014.

Superintendent of Documents, US Government Printing Office, Washington, DC 20402.

Arthritis Foundation, 3400 Peachtree Road, NE, Atlanta, GA 30326.

American Cancer Society, 777 Third Avenue, New York, NY 10017.

American Heart Association, 7320 Greenville Avenue, Dallas, TX 75231.

American Medical Association, Dept. of Food and Nutrition, 535 No. Dearborn Street, Chicago, IL 60610.

Society for Nutrition Education, 1736 Franklin Street, Oakland, CA 94612.

Alzheimer Disease and Related Disorders Association (ADRDA), 360 No. Michigan Ave., Chicago, IL 60601.

Administration on Aging/National Clearinghouse on Aging, US Dept. of Health and Human Services, Washington, DC 20201.

Deafness Research Foundation, Suite 705, 366 Madison Avenue, New York, NY 10017.

National Society for the Prevention of Blindness, Inc., 79 Madison Avenue, New York, NY 10801.

Parkinson's Disease Foundation, 107 Vista del Grande, San Carlos, CA 94070.

SAGE (Senior Actualization and Growth Explorations), 2455 Hilgard Avenue, Berkeley, CA 94709.

United Ostomy Association, 1111 Wilshire Boulevard, Los Angeles, CA 90017

American Association of Retired Persons/National Retired Teachers Association (AARP/NRTA), 1225 Connecticut Avenue, NW, Washington, DC 20036.

American Dietetic Association Gerontological Nutrition Practice Group, ADA,
    430 N. Michigan Avenue, Chicago, IL 60611.
American Geriatrics Society, 10 Columbus Circle, New York, NY 10019.
American Nursing Home Association, 1101 17th Street, NW, Washington, DC
    20045.
Grey Panthers, 3700 Chestnut Street, Philadelphia, PA 19104.

American Dental Association
211 East Chicago Avenue
Chicago, IL 60611

American Diabetes Association, Inc.
Two Park Avenue
New York, NY 10016

American Lung Association
1740 Broadway
New York, NY 10019

American Parkinson's Disease Association
116 John Street, Suite 417
New York, NY 10038

American Speech-Language-Hearing Association
10801 Rockville Pike
Rockville, MD 20852

Gerontological Society of America
Suite 305
1835 K Street NW
Washington, DC 20006

National Council on the Aging
600 Maryland Avenue SW, West Wing 100
Washington, DC 20024

National Heart, Lung, and Blood Institute
National Institutes of Health
9600 Rockville Pike
Building 31, Room 5A52
Bethesda, MD 20014

National Institute of Arthritis, Metabolism and Digestive Diseases
c/o Dr. George Brooks
Westwood Building, Room 637
Bethesda, MD 20014

National Kidney Foundation
Two Park Avenue
New York, NY 10016

Recording for the Blind, Inc.
215 East 58th Street
New York, NY 10022

Director, Bureau of Consumer Protection
Federal Trade Commission
Washington, DC 20580

Department of Housing and Urban Development
Division of Consumer Complaints
Washington, DC 20410

Health Care Financing Administration
Department of Health and Human Services
Washington, DC 20201

Division of Public Inquiries
Social Security Administration
6401 Security Boulevard
Baltimore, mD 21235

Veterans Administration
810 Vermont Avenue, NW
Washington, DC 20420

American Association of Retired Persons
1909 K Street NW
Washington, DC 20049

National Council of Senior Citizens
1511 K Street NW
Washington, DC 20005

National Association of Area Agencies on Aging
1828 L Street NW
Washington, DC 20036

Legal Services for the Elderly
132 West 43rd Street, 3rd Floor
New York, NY 10036

National Caucus and Center on Black Aged
1424 K Street NW
Suite 500
Washington, DC 20005

National Indian Council on Aging
P.O. Box 2088
Albuquerque, NM 87103

National Pacific-Asian Resource Center on Aging
618 Second Avenue
Suite 243
Seattle, WA 98104

Journals and Newsletters

ACSH News & Views. American Council on Science and Health, 1995 Broadway, New York, NY 10023.

National Council Against Health Fraud Newsletter. National Council Against Health Fraud, Inc., Box 1276 Loma Linda, CA 92354.

Nutrition Forum: A Monthly Newsletter. George F. Stickley Co. 210 W. Washington Square, Phila., PA 19106.

Environmental Nutrition. Environmental Nutrition, Inc., 52 Riverside Drive, Suite 15A, New York, NY 10024.

FDA Consumer. US Department of Health and Human Services/Food and Drug Administration, US Government Printing Office, Washington, DC 20402.

The Harvard Medical School Health Letter. 79 Garden Street, Cambridge, MA 02138.

Weight Control. Nutritional Management, Inc., 990 Washington St., Suite 211, Dedham, MA 02026.

Aging. Superintendent of Documents, Government Printing Office, Washington, DC 20402.

Geriatric Focus. Knoll Pharmaceutical Co., 386 Park Avenue South, New York, NY 10016.

Gerontopics. Publications Desk, New England Gerontology Center, 15 Garrison Avenue, Durham, NH 03824.

Journal of the American Geriatrics Society. American Geriatrics Society, 10 Columbus Circle, New York, NY 10019.

Modern Maturity. American Association of Retired Persons, 1225 Connecticut Avenue, NW, Washington, DC 20036.

The Journal of Gerontology. Gerontological Society, 1 Dupont Circle, Suite 520, Washington, DC 20036.

Audiovisuals:

"Food for Older Folks." Nasco, 901 Jamesville Avenue, Fort Atkinson, WI 53538.

"Food: More for Your Money." AHP, Inc., 9100 Sunset Boulevard, Los Angeles, CA 90069.

"Help Yourself to Better Health." Society for Nutrition Education, 1736 Franklin Street, Oakland, CA 94612.

"Nutrition Education for Older Americans." American Dietetic Association, 430 N. Michigan Avenue, Chicago, IL 60611 (cassette).

"The String Bean." McGraw-Hill Films/Association Films, Inc., 600 Grand Avenue, Ridgefield, NJ 07657.

INDEX